Renate Wernery · Ulrich Wernery · Jörg Kinne · Jaime Samour

Colour Atlas of Falcon Medicine

With collaboration of
Angel Luis Sánchez

schlütersche

Central Veterinary Research Laboratory, P.O. Box 597, Dubai, UAE
Fahad Bin Sultan Falcon Centre, P.O. Box 55, Riyadh 11322, Saudi Arabia
Falcon Center, Osterende 62, 27389 Helvesiek, Germany

Proofreading and translation assistance:
R. Scott Pirie BVM&S, Cert EP, Cert EM (Int. Med.), PhD, MRCVS

E-mail: info@schluetersche.de

Printed in Germany

ISBN 3-89993-007-X

Bibliographic information published by Die Deutsche Bibliothek

Die Deutsche Bibliothek lists this publication in the Deutsche Nationalbibliografie; detailed bibliographic data are available in the Internet at http://dnb.ddb.de.

2

Renate Wernery · Ulrich Wernery · Jörg Kinne · Jaime Samour

Colour Atlas of Falcon Medicine

Contents

Foreword

My first interest in birds of prey started over 20 years ago when an injured Tawny Owl was brought to me at the Central Veterinary Laboratory, Weybridge, England. The bird, which had a damaged wing and was suffering from hypothermia, had previously been taken to another establishment, but unfortunately they had no experience of working with raptors and suggested that it should be taken elsewhere. Fortunately the situation has improved significantly around the world and information on the care and treatment of raptors is now readily available to all those that have an interest in these magnificent birds by way of publications, conferences and of course the Internet.

The improved understanding and knowledge of raptor medicine and surgery during the past 20 years has resulted in a significant improvement in the health and hygiene of these birds. A major benefit of this has been the establishment of captive breeding programmes for some of the more endangered species of raptors with subsequent re-introduction back into their natural environment, the Mauritius Kestrel programme being a good example.

The generous financial support provided by individuals, charitable organisations, occasionally governments but above all the physical support of teams of enthusiastic people has led to significant advances in raptor biomedicine, particularly in the Middle East.

With dedicated institutes like the falcon hospitals in the United Arab Emirates and the Fahad bin Sultan Falcon Centre in the Kingdom of Saudi Arabia, research projects on raptor diseases, the development of new vaccines and the evaluation and efficacy of already instigated specific raptor vaccines can be undertaken. These well-equipped research establishments and specialist diagnostic centres are essential in the diagnosis of recognised and new and emerging diseases of raptors. In recent years diseases not previously recorded in these birds have emerged, and in an effort to try to counteract these sometimes fatal diseases, much needed research and good facilities are imperative. The popular perception of birds of prey is that as predators they are strong and resilient, as most raptor species are at the top of their food chain, however, those working with raptors know only too well that they are highly vulnerable to disease, contamination of the environment and changes to the ecosystem. In fact raptors generally are the barometers of how well we are managing our global environment.

The generous support of H.H. Gen. Sheikh Mohammed bin Rashid Al Maktoum and his brothers as well as the expertise and knowledge of the various contributing authors is well recognised. In particular those at the Central Veterinary Research Laboratory, Dubai who were responsible for initiating the production of this comprehensive work that has resulted in a publication that will make a significant contribution to expanding our knowledge and understanding of raptor biomedicine.

Ruth Manvell
Avian Virology, CVL,
Weybridge, Surrey, England

Preface

The objectives of the authors in publishing this book have been 2-fold:

Firstly, the Colour Atlas of Falcon Medicine is the logical follow-up of the »Color Atlas of Camelid Hematology« and secondly it enables the reader, veterinarians, falcon breeders and owners as well as laboratory technicians to utilize the knowledge of experienced scientists gained in decades of work with birds of prey.

It is furthermore the authors' anticipation to put the inclined reader into the position of broadening the capacity of their diagnostic tools by applying the contents of the eight following chapters of this book.

The first chapter serves as an introduction to falconry in the Middle East as it was introduced from the Arabian Peninsula to the noble courts of Frederick II and continues on into modern times.

One of the achievements in falconry in the 21st century in Arabia can be credited to Dubai's falconers who introduced the commendable practice of flying falcons in accordance with CITES regulations, instead of birds taken from the wild. It is hoped that this serves as an exemplary practice to other countries with a history of falconry. All species of the family *Falconidae* (falcons) are listed in the CITES Appendices I and II, which makes it compulsory for all falcon owners to possess a CITES permit to enter or leave a country. Strict regulations have also now been implemented by the United Arab Emirates authorities. All birds, either purchased abroad or bred in the U.A.E. must be registered with the U.A.E. CITES Management Authority.

The second chapter revolves around haematology and blood chemistry of birds of prey. Meticulous effort went into the establishment of haematological reference values of 7 different clinically normal falcon and hybrid species. For blood chemistry values the latest technology available has been applied. However, it should be emphasized that it is extremely difficult to obtain »normal« haematological and biochemistry values for falcons. Both, handling stress during restraint and delays in analyses following the sampling procedure, can result in significant alterations in certain parameters.

The authors would like to take the opportunity to create awareness within the medical suppliers' industry for the need for new technological developments. This would include an automated system for the differentiation of avian leucocytes, and blood chemistry analyses which could be performed on low blood volumes usually obtained following venopuncture in this species. Additionally, through the creation of this atlas, it is the authors' sincere desire to stimulate scientists worldwide to shed more light on the role and importance of blood chemistry in the various falcon diseases.

The following six chapters cover viral, bacterial, fungal, parasitic, miscellaneous and undiagnosed diseases, focussing on the most significant signs and alterations found in clinical presentations, gross-pathology and histopathology. The reader may also appreciate an additional insight into some diseases of the food animals for birds of prey.

For an improved understanding of the mentioned diseases, the authors volunteered to demonstrate alterations in haematological and blood biochemical values in sick falcons. In order to provide a more detailed understanding of the various diseases described in each chapter, the authors have included both the haematological and blood biochemical profiles associated with each disease.

This book offers an extensive coverage of the most prevalent diseases occurring in falcons. Consequently, the authors consider this text to provide a valuable diagnostic overview to all individuals who love and admire this graceful, swift and noble bird and the art of hunting which has brought joy and happiness over the course of centuries.

Renate Wernery
Ulrich Wernery
Jörg Kinne
Jaime Samour

Acknowledgements

The authors are deeply indebted to His Highness Sheikh Mohamed Bin Rashid Al Maktoum, Minister of Defence of the United Arab Emirates for his generous contribution to financing the publication of this book, and for having the foresight to establish the Central Veterinary Research Laboratory, where all laboratory analyses on falcons were conducted.

The authors gratefully acknowledge the cooperation, help and advice from Dr. Ali Ridha, the Administrative Director of the Central Veterinary Research Laboratory in Dubai.

Very special efforts have been contributed by the CVR Laboratory staff: Mrs. Shirley Korah, Mrs. Sunitha Joseph, Mrs. Reena Zachariah, Mrs. R. Mareena George, Mrs. Tina Ostwald, Mrs. Kate Koranyi, Mrs. Marina Joseph, Mr. Yousuf Abubaker, Prof. R. Schuster, Dr. Peter Nagy, Dr. Jutka Juhasz, Mr. C. Vishwanatan, Mr. Rajan Babu without their help we could never have completed this work.

Sincere thanks are expressed to the veterinarians who work for the Ruling Family of Dubai, Dr. Alok Sharma at the Emirates Falcon Hospital and Dr. Peter McKinney at the Al Safa Falcon Hospital, as well as to the veterinarians at the Dubai Falcon Hospital, Dr. Antonio di Somma and Dr. Tom Bailey and Dr. Laszlo Molnar for their support. Many thanks also go to the sponsors of the Fahad Bin Sultan Falcon Centre in Saudi Arabia and the Abu Dhabi Falcon Hospital. Their contributions and submission of specimens were invaluable.

Sincere thanks are extended to Mr. Harald Küspert and his Falcon Center in Germany for donating falcons for different experiments and allowing us to conduct herpes vaccine trials on his falcons.

Last, but not least the authors are particularly grateful to Mrs. Ruth Manvell, Avian Virology, CVL, Weybridge, Surrey, England and her team for identifying and serotyping the viral strains.

Dubai, summer 2003

Renate Wernery
Ulrich Wernery
Jörg Kinne
Jaime Samour

Chapter 1

Falcons and Falconry in the Middle East

Falcons and falconry have formed an integral part of life in the deserts of the Middle East since ancient times. In the old days, weary Bedouins on camel back used to toil for days through the sun-scorched sands of the Arabian Peninsula using falcons in search of quarry to supplement their basic diet. In those days, falconry was both sustainable and a subsistence form of hunting. In modern times, falconry is still very popular throughout the Gulf countries and it is considered a sport. Yet, to Arabs, falconry is an opportunity to go back to the desert where they once belonged and to reunite with a way of life that is already gone. Fast-cars and fast-food restaurants, in a fast-changing world, are a constant threat to local customs and traditions, but falconry remains deeply rooted in the hearts of the Arab people as a way of communion with the past.

In the old days, Bedouins used to trap, train and hunt with passage falcons. These were subsequently released at the end of the season, as the caring of birds throughout the year could strain their already limited resources. Today after the hunting season, Arab falconers keep their falcons in air-conditioned rooms or in free-flying aviaries during the long moulting months, so they can be used again for the following season. As a byproduct of this change of attitude, a substantially large population of hunting falcons are kept in captivity every year throughout the Gulf countries. The number of falcons used for falconry in the Middle East has been estimated to be as high as 8,000 to 10,000 falcons. The need for professional health care to such a large captive population of falcons prompted the establishment of modern falcon hospitals in most countries of the region. In this respect, there are falcon veterinary facilities run by professional veterinarians in Qatar, Bahrain but, especially, in the United Arab Emirates and the Kingdom of Saudi Arabia. In addition, many modern falconry hunting parties from the Gulf States, take their own veterinarians and technicians in order to provide veterinary services to hunting falcons in field clinics fitted within camp tents or custom built and fully-equipped caravans.

Arab falconry is literally as full of customs and traditions as the Arab falconers themselves. Falcons in the Middle East are still selected and valued by the measurements of the total length of the wing and the girth around the shoulders and the colour of the plumage. Falcons are still fitted with the same type of falconry furniture, following the same pattern, as the ones designed in ancient times. Falconers still train falcons using a lure made of bustards' wings tied up in a bundle as it was done by their forefathers. The favourite quarry remains to be the elusive and well-camouflaged Houbara Bustard (*Chlamydotis undulata*), but also the Stone Curlew (*Burhinus oedicnemus*) and the Cape Hare (*Lepus capensis*) are favoured to a lesser extent. The courage and determination of a falcon lives on in songs and poetry. Yes, till today, the Arab falconer is involved in an intrinsic affair with his falcons, exactly as it was more than two thousand years ago.

The most common falcon species used for falconry in the Middle East includes the Saker falcon (*Falco cherrug*), the Peregrine falcon (*Falco peregrinus*), the Lanner falcon (*Falco biarmicus*), the Barbary falcon (*Falco pelegrinoides*) the Gyr falcon (*Falco rusticolus*) and different hybrids. A ban on the import of wild-caught falcons took effect in 2002 in the United Arab Emirates, therefore only captive bred birds are allowed into the country to be used in the sport of falconry. Other countries may follow. This will ease the pressure on free-living falcons, particularly in the Central Asian region.

Veterinary medicine has made a significant impact on falcons and falconry in the Middle East over the past 10 years. A handful of veterinarians have persevered in pioneering techniques and therapeutic regimes to combat the most important diseases and medical conditions in the region. The most difficult aspect of veterinary work with falcons in the Middle East is how to deal with deeply-rooted ancestral convictions and practices. Public awareness through educational and promotional campaigns may prove most effective in the long term in controlling and hopefully eradicating some of the main medical complaints affecting falcons.

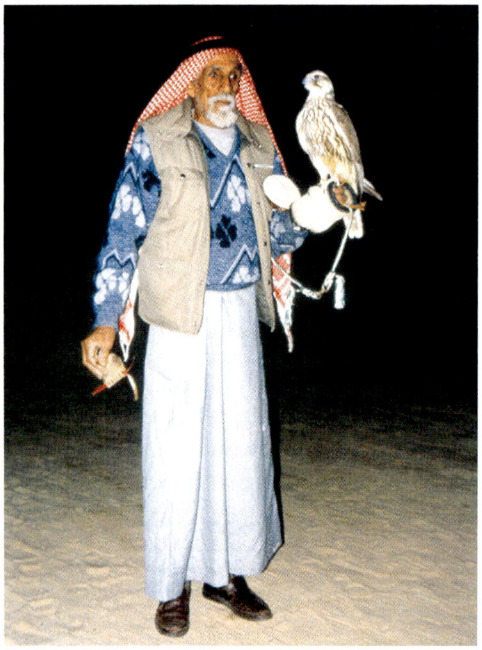

Figure 1.1: In the Middle East, falconers learn the art of falconry from their fathers and grandfathers, as this wealth of information is conferred from generation to generation as a legacy of pride and honour.

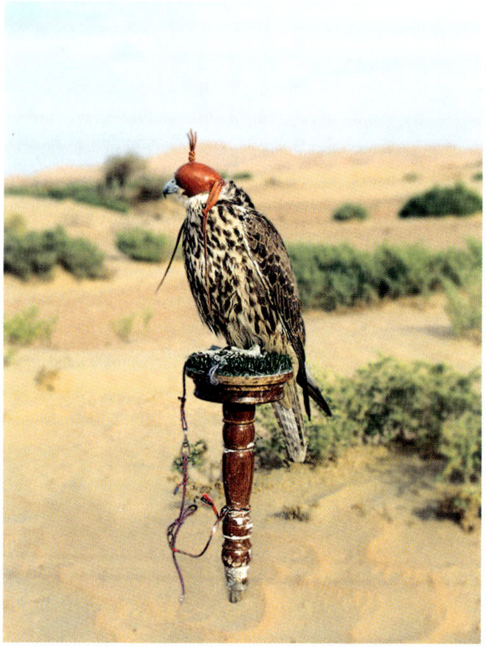

Figure 1.2: Falcons and falconry have formed an integral part of life in the desert since ancient times. Arabian scholars have been able to establish that falconry in the Arabian Peninsula saw its early beginnings during pre-Islamic times in the Al Jaheliya era with Al Harith bin Muawiyah bin Thor bin Kindah.

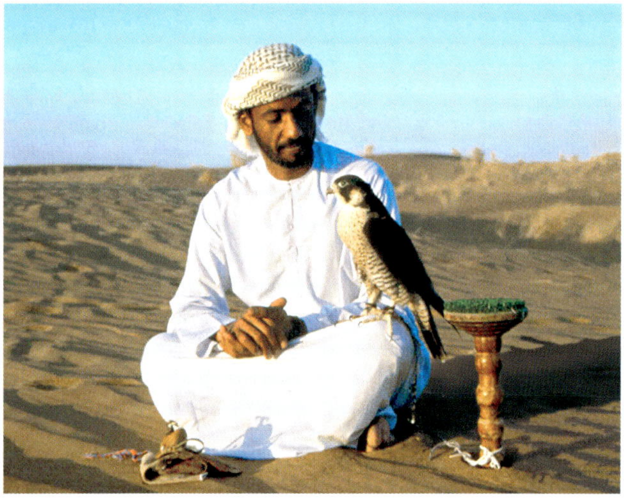

Figure 1.3: The taming of a falcon demands great patience, complete devotion and a deep knowledge of psychology. Essentially, the falconer has to gradually build a close relationship with his falcon. Yet, this relationship is not the type associated with a master and a servant, but a partnership between two faithful and loyal friends: A relationship based on trust and understanding.

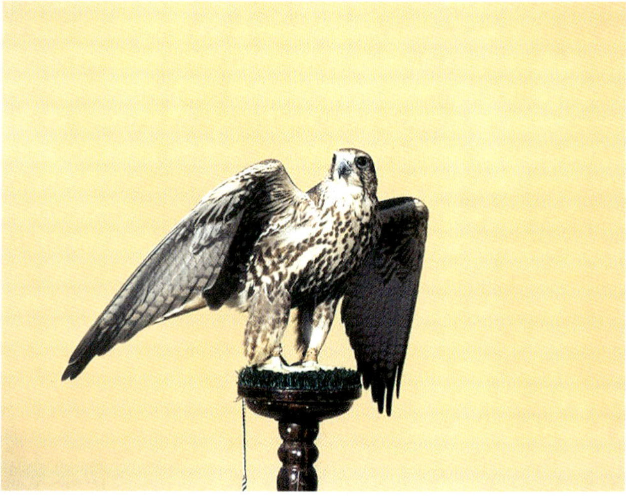

Figure 1.4: The Saker falcon (*Falco cherrug*) has been the favourite falcon amongst Arabs in the skilful art of falconry for centuries. Arab falconers have traditionally favoured this species on account of its remarkable endurance in flight, great strength and the ability to cope with the rigorous environment of the deserts of the Arabian Peninsula.

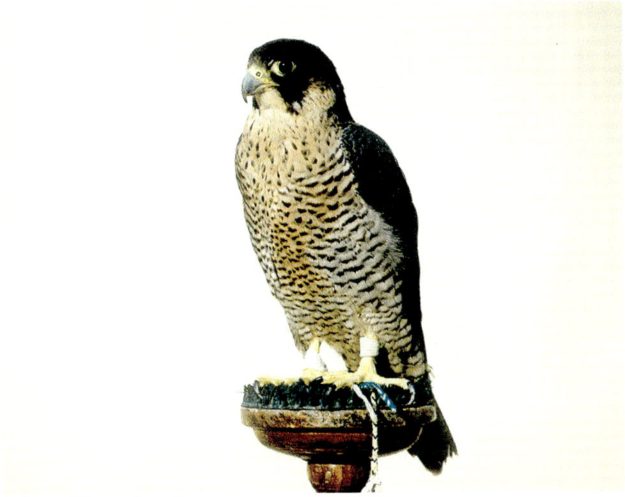

Figure 1.5: The Peregrine falcon (*Falco peregrinus*) is without a doubt the »Prince of the Falcons«. Its beauty, grace and extraordinary speed are legendary amongst falconers from all around the world. In the Middle East however, the Peregrine falcon occupies only second place amongst the favourite species used in Arab falconry. The name in Arabic given to the peregrine is »Al Shaheen« which is an expression derived from the Persian language meaning »balance«.

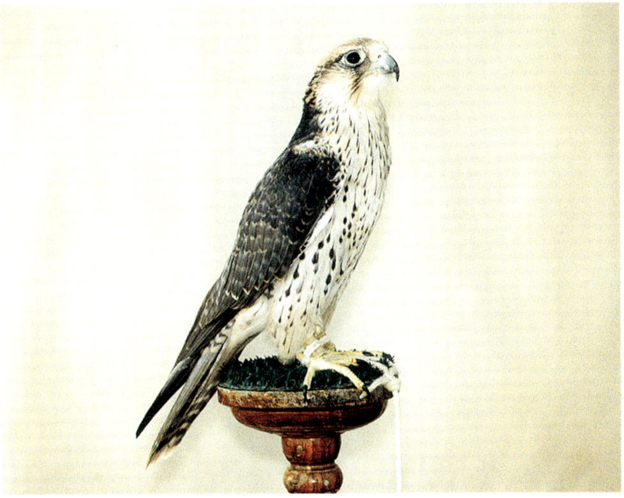

Figure 1.6: The Lanner falcon (*Falco biarmicus*) is a large desert falcon and yet another favourite species used in falconry in the Middle East. However, most experienced Arab falconers consider Lanners as falcons for beginners as they lack the qualities of the ideal falcon to hunt large quarry such as Houbara Bustards.

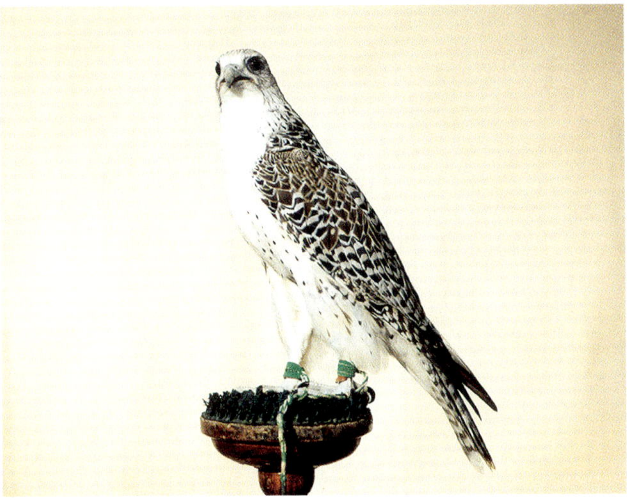

Figure 1.7: The Gyr falcon (*Falco rusticolus*) is the largest falcon in the world and a species that is highly valued in Arab falconry. It's large size and great strength made Gyrs greatly favoured during the early 70's, but their popularity soon waned when it was realised that they were not able to cope with the extreme weather conditions prevalent in the Middle East. Surprisingly, Gyr falcons are now back in even larger numbers than ever before. This is probably due to the breakdown of the Soviet Union and the desire of falcon traders within the emerging republics to open new markets with countries in the Middle East.

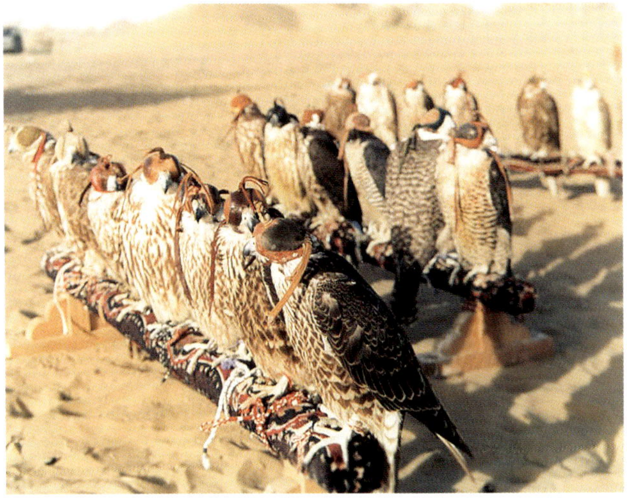

Figure 1.8: A large group of primarily Gyr hybrid falcons during a hunting trip. A hybrid falcon is the product of a cross between two different species of falcons. This is achieved under captive conditions and by the use of artificial insemination (AI) techniques. The production of hybrid falcons was initiated during the early 70's across the United States and Europe. Nowadays, hybrid falcons are produced mainly in Canada, United States, Germany and the United Kingdom to supply the demand across the world. More recently, two captive breeding centres have been established in the United Arab Emirates to produce hybrid falcons for local use.

1

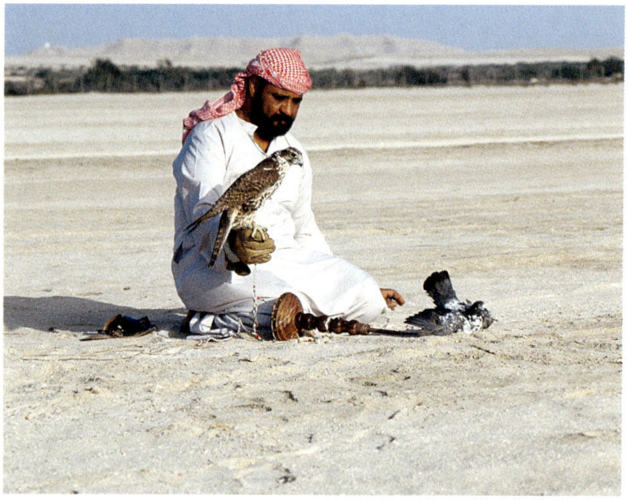

Figure 1.9: A falconer presenting a live pigeon to a novice falcon during the first stages of training. The pigeon is secured with a short line from the stand to one of its legs to prevent escape. The falcon is usually encouraged by the falconer using a series of characteristic vocalizations to jump and kill the pigeon.

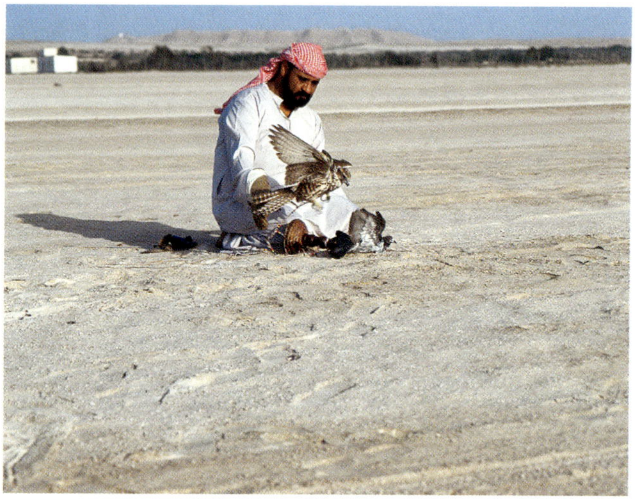

Figure 1.10: The same falcon taking a short jump to make a kill. Even though it appears a small step, this short jump represents one significant step forward in the training process of the falcon.

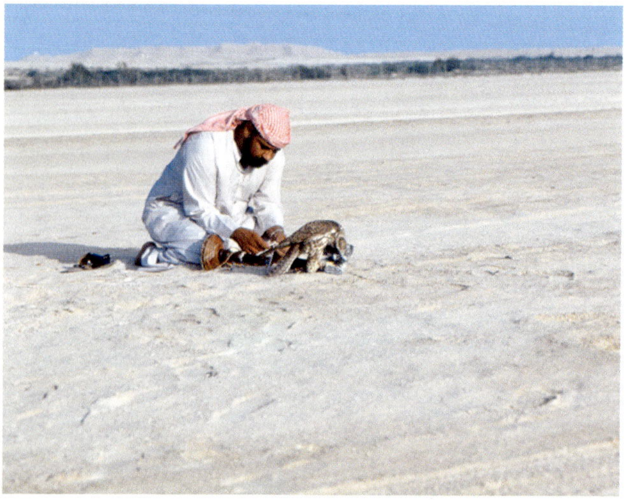

Figure 1.11: The falcon has made the kill and is actively eating. The falconer kneels besides the bird calling and vocalizing to encourage the falcon to eat.

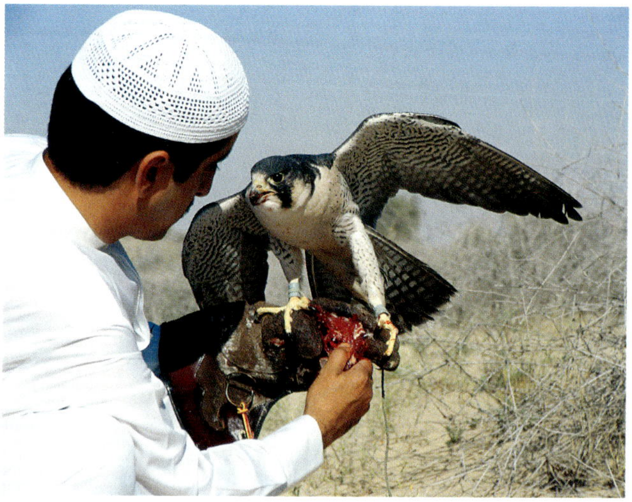

Figure 1.12: The falcon and its prey are both gently lifted off the ground, and the falcon is encouraged to eat on the wrist of the falconer. This helps building up the trust between falconer and falcon.

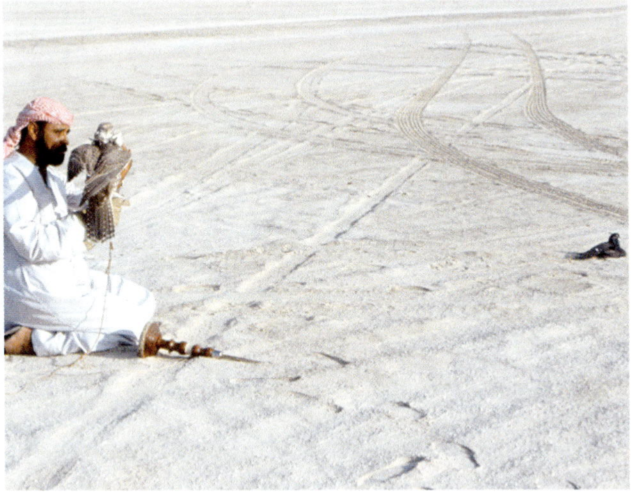

Figure 1.13: In a more advanced stage of training the falcon is persuaded to take a short flight from the wrist of the falconer to catch and kill a pigeon placed a few meters away.

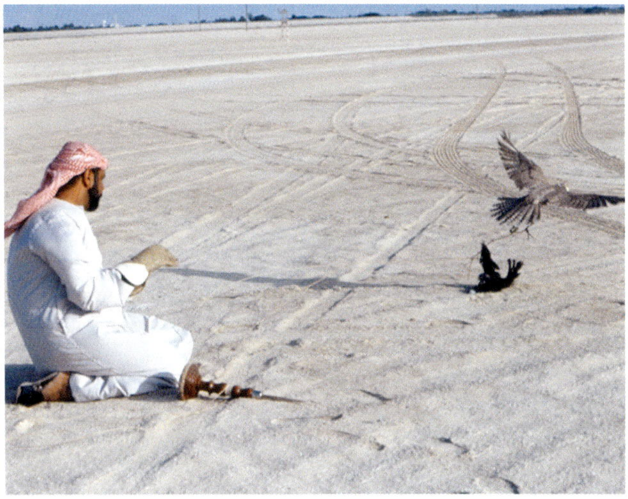

Figure 1.14: The falcon making a pass over the pigeon as it miscalculated the distance. The falcon in this case landed a short distance away and had to return to the pigeon to kill it. This incident tends to happen very often with novice birds and all form part of the training process.

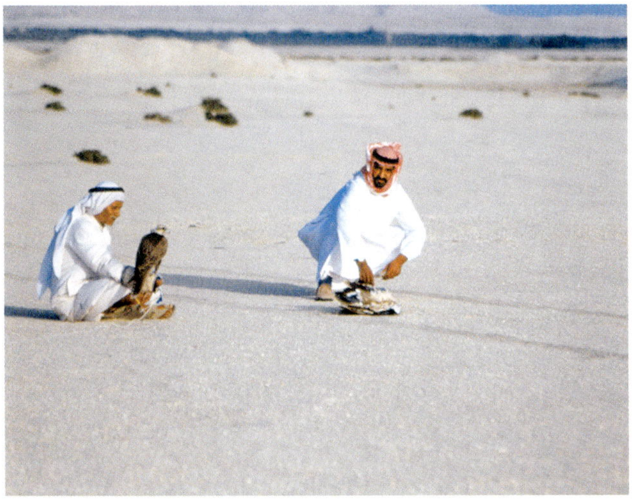

Figure 1.15: Introducing a novice falcon to the lure. Typically the Arabian lure is made up of one or two pairs of Houbara Bustard wings tied up together in a bundle. Commonly a piece of meat is attached to the lure to reward the falcon for catching it. Lures are designed to introduce the falcon to the colour and colouration pattern of the wing of its prey.

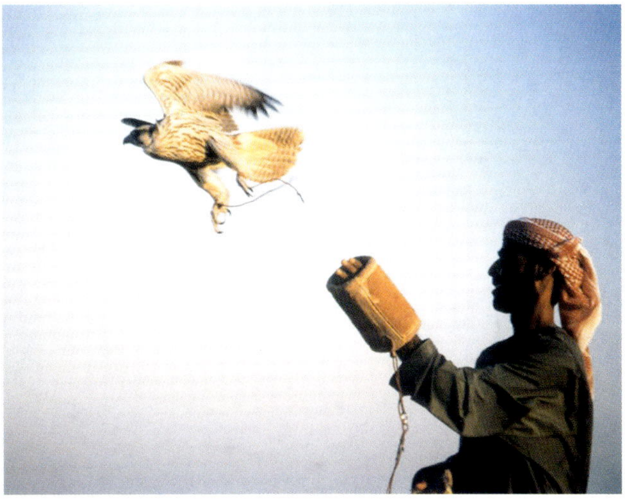

Figure 1.16: In a more advanced stage of training, the falcon is released and is allowed to fly free to a calling falconer positioned at a distance of 600 or 800 m. This second falconer usually calls the falcon while swinging a pigeon or a lure. This stage is crucial and there are no short cuts. The falconer simply has to assess whether the falcon is ready to fly freely or not. An impatient falconer and a premature judgement will inevitably result in failure with the falcon and all the falconers' efforts disappearing.

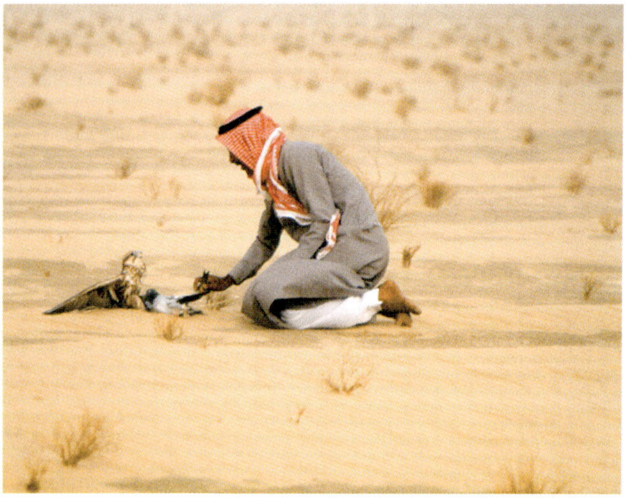

Figure 1.17: Throughout the training period, the falconer has to be patient and understanding with his falcon. It is never a good idea to accelerate any stage of training or to try to hurry the falcon to do something the falcon is still not prepared to do. The breaking up of the bond between falcon and falconer during any stage of the training process consequently results in delays and frustration.

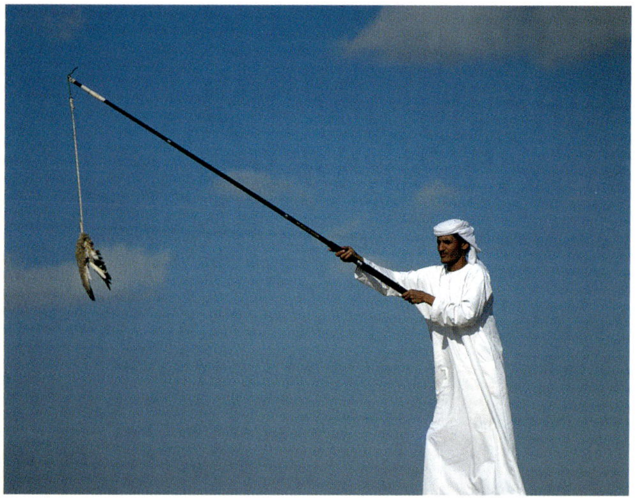

Figure 1.18: In some countries of the region, falconers use poles (fishing rods are ideal) to attach the lure using a short stout rope. The lure will be swung in circles while the falconer calls loudly to attract the attention of the falcon. When the falcon is close to the lure, this is swiftly moved in a continuous graceful circular movement. The same routine is usually executed 5 to 10 times, until the lure is deposited on the ground allowing the falcon to catch it. This practice is repeated up to two times daily increasing the number of passes up to 25 to 30.

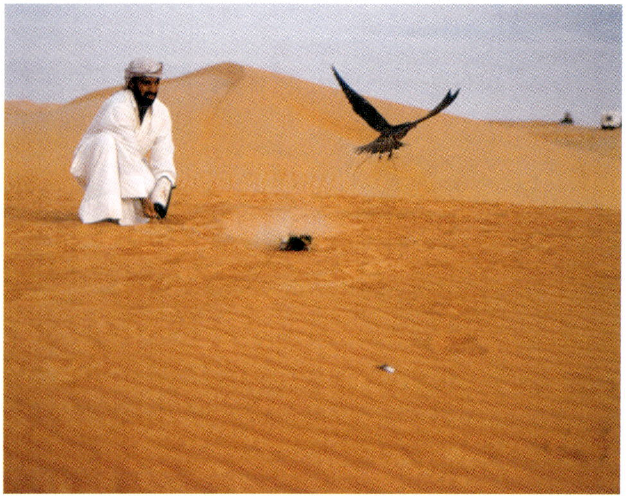

Figure 1.19: A falcon in the process of passing over the lure after having failed to catch it. Some falconers prefer their falcons to catch the lure up in the air, since this minimises the danger of breaking feathers on the ground. Falcons trained using lures are fit and have great stamina, permitting them to confront more effectively the challenges of the hunting season.

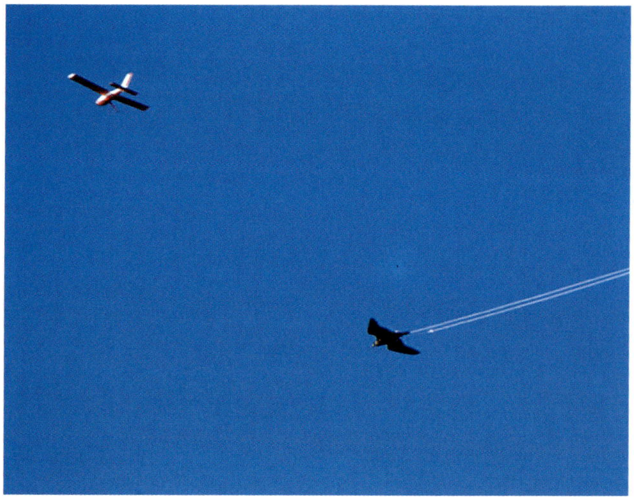

Figure 1.20: Modern training of a falcon: A dead prey, usually a quail, is fixed at a string attached to a remote controlled plane. The exercise for the falcon can be very strenuous as the plane can increase its speed at will. Depending on the stamina of the bird, the hunt may last 15 to 20 minutes. At the end, the plane slows down, the falcon catches the quarry, and the rope is hooked off the plane (courtesy M. Martin).

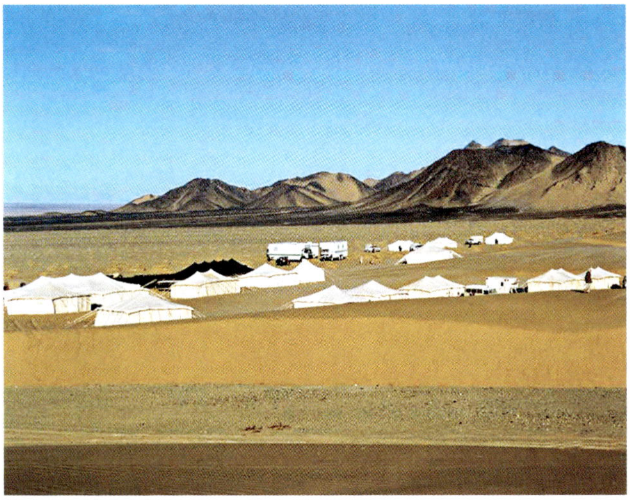

Figure 1.21: Modern Arab falconry hunting trips are a way of social life, in which members of one or two families or a group of friends go out together for a few days. However, the hunting parties of members of the Royal Families can be very large. The complexity of these parties are directly related to who and how important the host is, bringing together members of families and friends for a day spent in the desert in the traditional way of the forefathers.

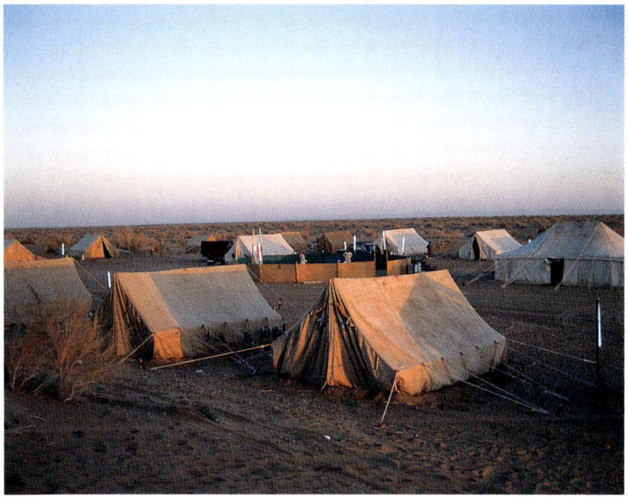

Figure 1.22: A hunting camp showing an open sitting room or »ennah«. In the old days, the ennah was an enclosure created by the use of natural dry bushes to form a low wall. The purpose of this was to create a barrier against the wind and cold weather. A modern ennah, such as the one in the picture, is made of canvas and the use of poles. Commonly a fire is lit at the centre and falconers sit on carpets all around to recount the happenings of the day.

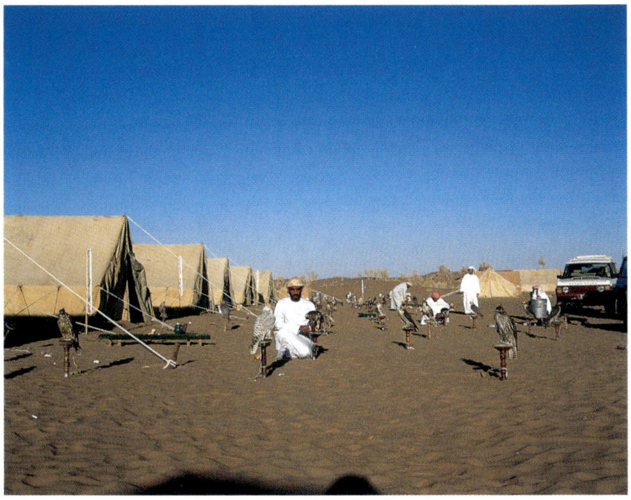

Figure 1.23: A general view of the weathering area for falcons of a hunting camp. The tents are intended for housing the falcon keepers so they can provide constant supervision to the falcons and tend to their needs.

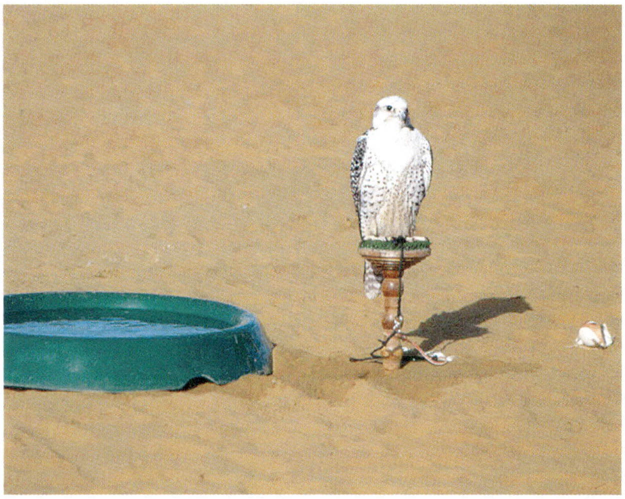

Figure 1.24: Water basins should also be provided for falcons, in particular to Peregrines, Gyr and Gyr hybrids to take a bath. In addition, spraying falcons with water, to help them cope with the midday heat, is also a good idea and most falconers do this routinely.

1

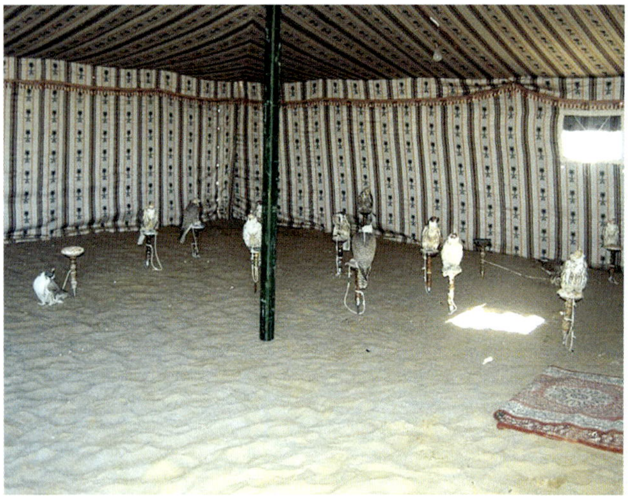

Figure 1.25: During hunting trips it is highly recommended to include some extra tents for the falcons. The ideal type is square tents measuring 5 m x 5 m provided with windows and doors. One of these tents can easily accommodate 8 to 10 hooded falcons overnight to protect them from the cold, rain and sandstorms. During the day, the windows and doors of these tents can be opened and provide an ideal shelter for falcons from the baking sun.

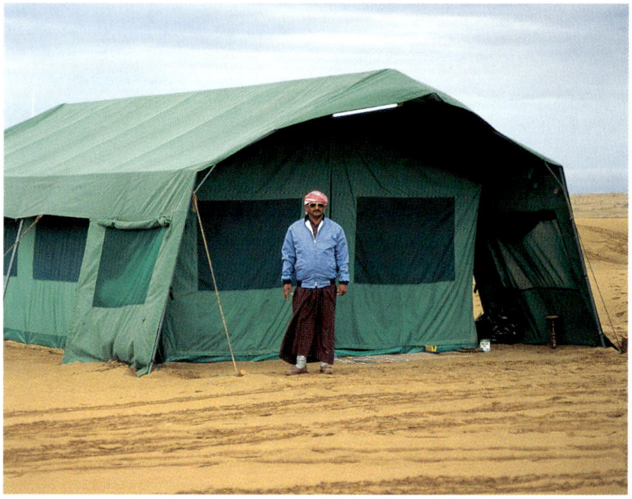

Figure 1.26: Nowadays, many large hunting parties take along field falcon hospitals to attend to common veterinary problems encountered during hunting trips. The tent shown here is a light weight unit mounted on an aluminium frame. The inner tent is provided with a rubberized floor, a main front door and several windows fitted with mosquito netting. The door and windows are provided with Velcro® fasteners and zippers to exclude dust and sand during windy days. The outer skin provides thermal insulation during extreme hot weather.

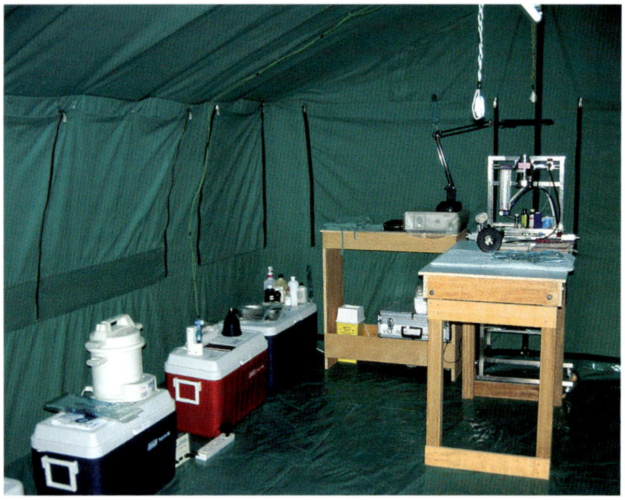

Figure 1.27: An internal view of the field hospital shown in the previous photograph. Basic furniture includes an examination table and a side table for the placement of equipment and instruments. Both tables are made of lightweight wood with Formica® tops and provided with legs on hinges that can be folded underneath. The equipment and materials are placed over the same cool boxes and crates that are originally used to transport them. Basic equipment includes anaesthetic machine, portable autoclave, endoscopy unit and equipment, microscope, electrocautery unit, complete surgical instrument set and hospital and clinical consumables.

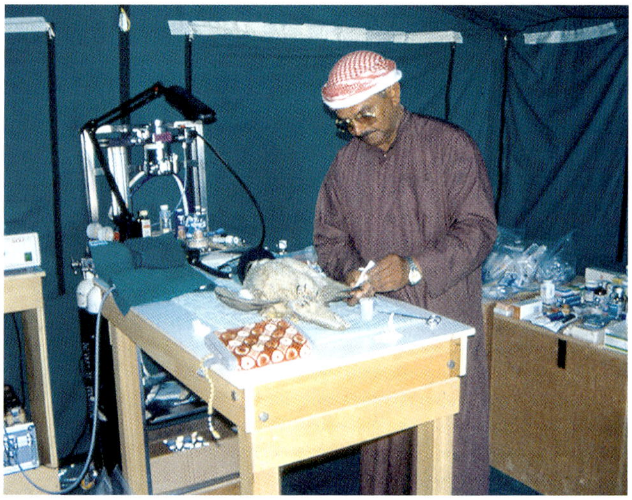

Figure 1.28: A falcon technician within the field hospital in the process of examining the feathers of a falcon. In hunting falcons, the integrity of the primary and tail feathers is of the utmost importance for flight performance. Invariably, feathers tend to get damaged during inadequate handling and transport, crash and fighting accidents or while pursuing quarry. »Imping«, an old medieval term widely used by falconers, is the art of repairing fractured or bent feathers. This is probably the most common problem encountered during hunting trips.

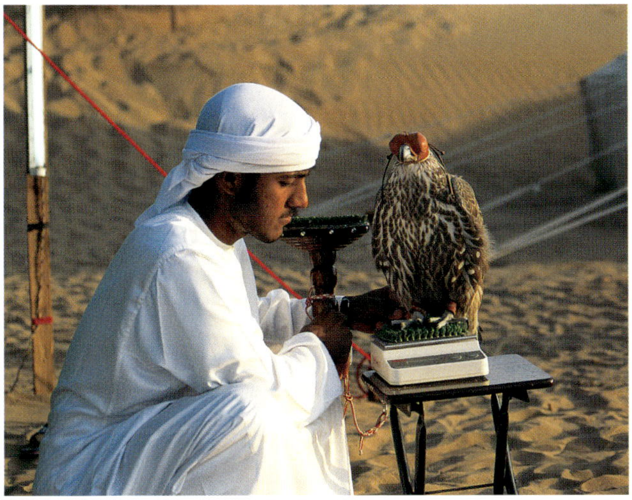

Figure 1.29: During hunting trips, the bodyweight of each falcon should be closely monitored in order to maintain its hunting ability. The weight of each falcon should be taken each day in the morning and soon after casting. This young falconer is using an electronic scale to weigh his falcon during a hunting trip.

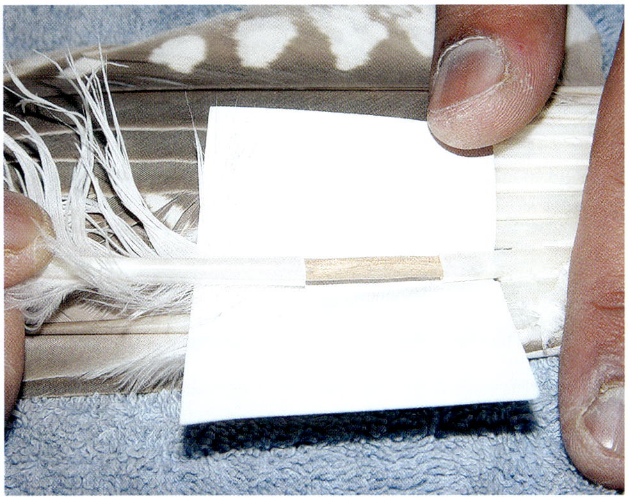

Figure 1.30: Total feather replacement is indicated when the feather is fractured at the proximal section of the feather shaft. The fractured feather is cut approximately 15 mm to 25 mm from the skin using a nail cutter. The new feather is placed in position to assess the length making sure to maintain bilateral symmetry with the opposite wing. A bamboo peg, about 80 to 100 mm long, is prepared by sharpening both ends to match loosely the diameter of the shaft of the new feather and the empty shaft of the wing. The wooden peg is firstly glued into the shaft of the new feather using fast setting epoxy glue. Additional glue is then placed into the shaft of the wing making sure the feather is properly aligned. A small cardboard card should be placed under the imping site to prevent glue from smearing adjacent feathers. The wing should then be closed in the natural anatomical position and all the feathers held in place using hair fasteners until the glue is set.

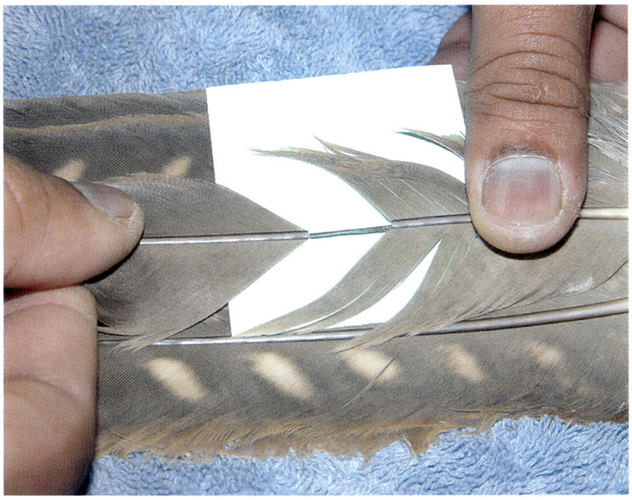

Figure 1.31: Partial feather replacement is indicated if the fracture has occurred at the mid-shaft or at the distal end of the feather. If the fracture is complete and the feather fragment is missing, a similar fragment must be procured from an identical feather. Conversely, the fragment may still be present and attached to the rest of the feather and can be used. Therefore, in both cases the ends of the fragments are left out using a fine-pointed scissor and a fine nail file. A previously prepared imping needle of a suitable length and diameter is carefully inserted on both fragments to make a narrow channel. The needle is then fixed onto the fragment and the rest of the feather using a small amount of methacrylate glue.

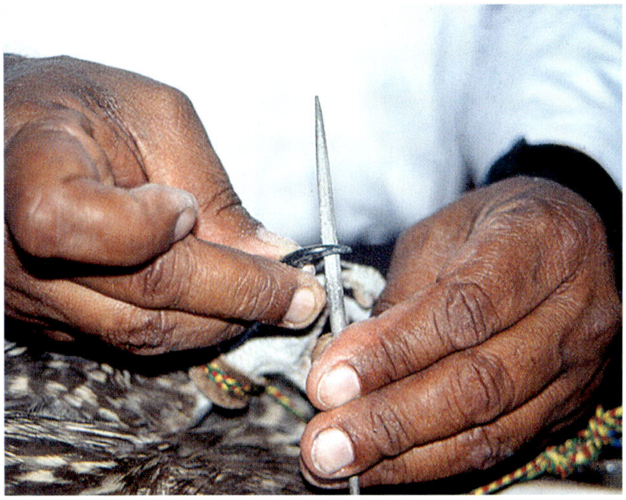

Figure 1.32: »Coping« is an old medieval term meaning the trimming and re-shaping of talons and beak. Overgrown talons are best trimmed using a guillotine-type nail cutter. The talon is then re-shaped using a sharp blade and nail files. The use of a lanolin or paraffin based hand cream is recommended after trimming and reshaping of the talons. Ideally, falcons should have the talons trimmed before placing them into moulting chambers.

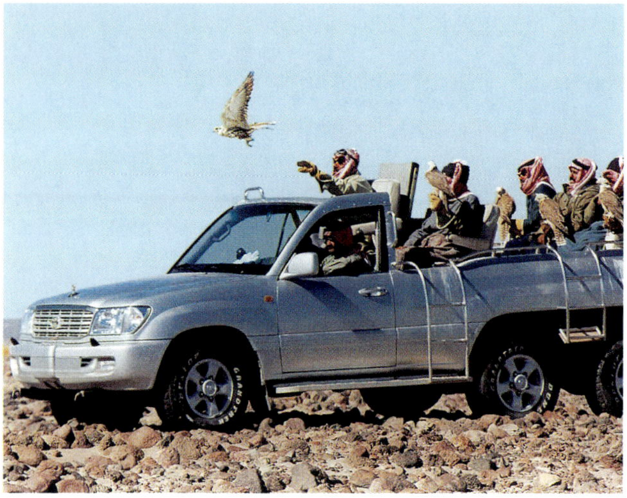

Figure 1.33: A hunting party is usually integrated by a group of 6 to 8 falconers in 3 to 4 cars driving across the sands. Commonly, there is a leading car carrying an expert tracker. He will be looking for the characteristic footprints of the Houbara Bustard impressed on the fine sand. When tracks are found, a »spotter« falcon is taken out of the car, its hood is removed so it can scan the ground in front of the vehicles. When the »spotter« falcon sees a Houbara and locks on it, a second falcon is released and the chase begins.

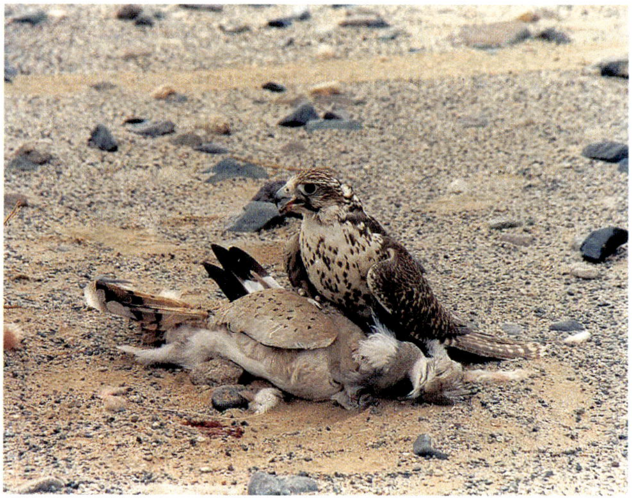

Figure 1.34: A saker falcon holding firmly the Houbara Bustard that had just caught. Immediately after making the kill, the falcon will start pecking the neck in order to severe the head. This is carried out by instinct to make sure the prey is truly dead. The falcon will then proceed to pluck some feathers from the chest and start eating actively.

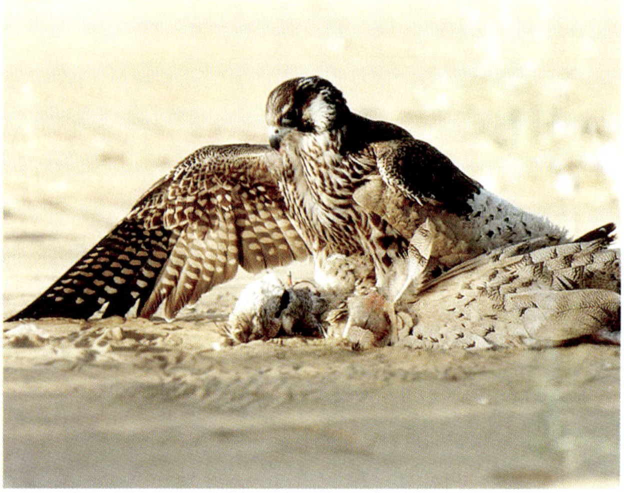

Figure 1.35: Peregrine falcons are much smaller birds than Gyr and Saker falcons. However, a female Peregrine weighing 700 to 800 g would normally engage and kill a much heavier Houbara Bustard weighing up to 2000 g. Peregrine falcons favour catching prey in mid-air sometimes at a very high altitude.

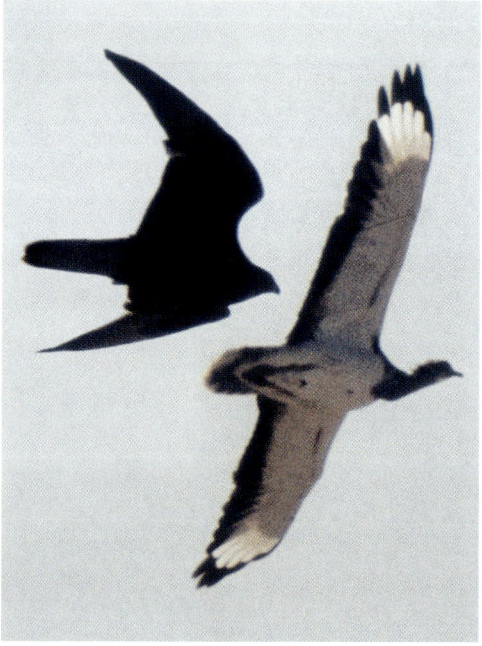

Figure 1.36: A Gyr x Saker hybrid chasing a Houbara Bustard.

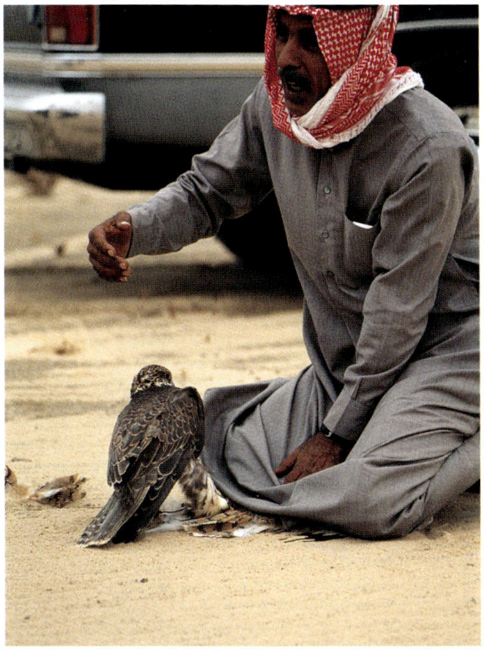

Figure 1.37: A Saker falcon had just caught a Houbara Bustard. The falconer is covering the live Houbara using his dress and is asking to be brought a dead pigeon to deceive the falcon and retrieve the live Houbara. Houbara Bustards rescued in this way are kept and will later be used for training a novice falcon.

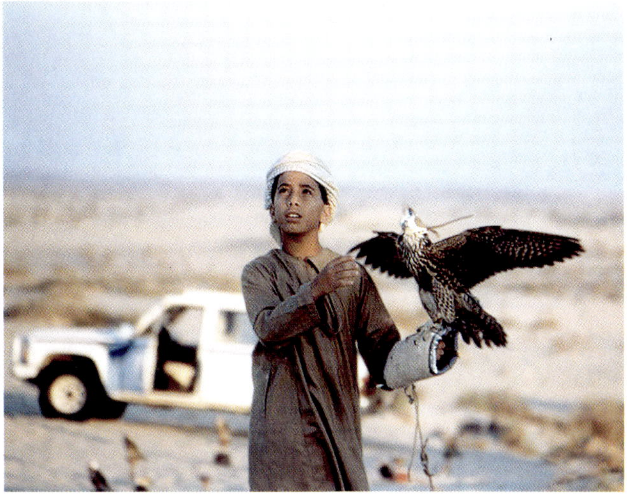

Figure 1.38: »Hunting is part of civilised man's life and no community should be deprived of the opportunity to indulge in it. If, however, it is going to lead to the extinction of the animals hunted it must be moderated lest new generations should one day find themselves the only species of animal left on the Earth« (Abdullah Nuwais, 1976, Undersecretary of the Ministry of Information and Culture, Abu Dhabi, United Arab Emirates).

2

Chapter 2

Haematology and blood biochemistry

The use of laboratory tests as an aid to the diagnosis of clinical disease has become commonplace in avian practice. However, it is important to realize the limitations of laboratory results. There is no substitute for a thorough clinical examination, and therefore clinicians should realize that clinical pathology should always be regarded as an ancillary diagnostic aid.

The analysis of avian blood samples has become a routine part of diagnostic evaluation and research. It is useful in the diagnosis of clinical disease, performance monitoring, pre-anaesthetic checks and pre-purchase examinations. Additionally, certain tests may be required for insurance purposes and import/export requirements.

Method for blood sample collection

The total blood volume in clinically normal birds is in the range of 6 ml–11 ml per 100 g of bodyweight. Thus, a falcon weighing 950 g would have approximately 57 ml–104.5 ml of blood of which, in a clinically normal individual, up to 10 % (5.7 ml–10.4 ml), can be safely withdrawn without having any detrimental effect on the patient. However, only 0.2 ml–0.3 ml of blood is generally sufficient to carry out a comprehensive haematology examination in a falcon, when manual methods are used. For automated methodology including haematology and biochemistry, a minimum amount of 2.0 ml to 3.0 ml of blood is required.

In falcons, blood samples are commonly collected using the basilic vein (*Vena cutanea ulnaris superficialis)* (Figure 2.1 a). In addition, other preferred sites include the right jugular vein (*Vena jugularis dextra*) (Figure 2.1 b), as this is generally larger than the left in most avian species, and the caudal tibial vein (*Vena metatarsalis plantaris superficialis*) (Figure 2.1 c).

The authors recommend obtaining blood samples from a basilic vein while the falcon is cast on its back. The preferred materials for venipuncture include a 23 or 25 gauge disposable needle, bent from the base at approximately 25° angle and a 1 ml or 3 ml disposable syringe. In falcons the optimal area for collecting a blood sample from a basilic vein is along the medial section of the vein. The preferred side is from the right wing if you are right handed, while the left wing would be the preferred side if you are left handed. Venipuncture immediately above the elbow joint is not recommended, as haemostasis is difficult to achieve at this site in most cases. The application of digital pressure with the thumb at the proximal humerus would help raising the vein, making it clearly visible running parallel to the external aspect of the humerus. After separating the feathers and preparing the site with an alcohol swab, the bent needle is gently inserted into the vein at an approximately 45° angle. The sample can now be collected taking precaution not to exert high negative pressure while withdrawing with the syringe since this will invariably result in the collapse of the vein. While withdrawing the sample, it is recommended to continue maintaining pressure on the proximal humerus to ensure a raised and well-defined vein. It is essential to avoid sudden movements that can alarm the bird and trigger a struggle, as this can easily lacerate the vein and result in a haematoma or, what is worse, a severe haemorrhage.

After collection, a small ball of dry cotton wool should be placed over the venipuncture site and the wing closed to maintain pressure over the site for a few seconds. It is strongly advisable to check the venipuncture site before releasing the bird back to its enclosure to make sure no post collection haemorrhage has occurred.

After blood collection, the EDTA or heparin tubes are gently shaken to avoid blood clots and/or haemolysis. Reject any sample that contains clots or is haemolysed, as the processing of such samples would invariably lead to inaccurate and, therefore, misleading results.

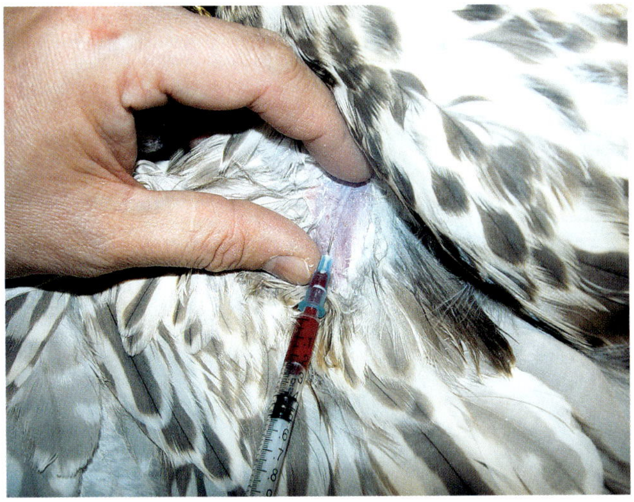

Figure 2.1 a: Blood sampling from a basilic vein (*Vena cutanea ulnaris superficialis*).

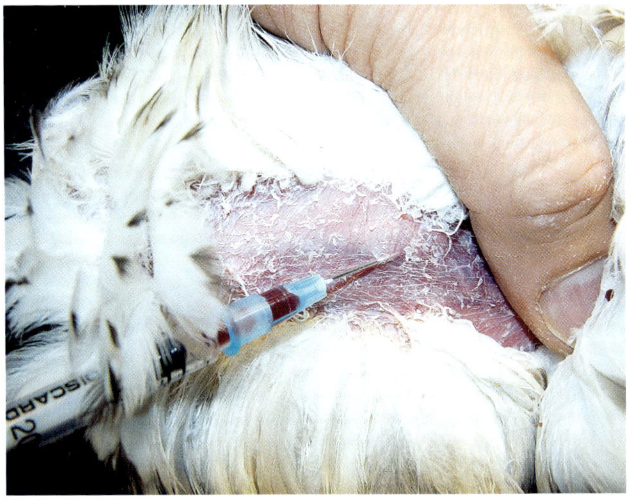

Figure 2.1 b: Blood sampling from the right jugular vein (*Vena jugularis dextra*).

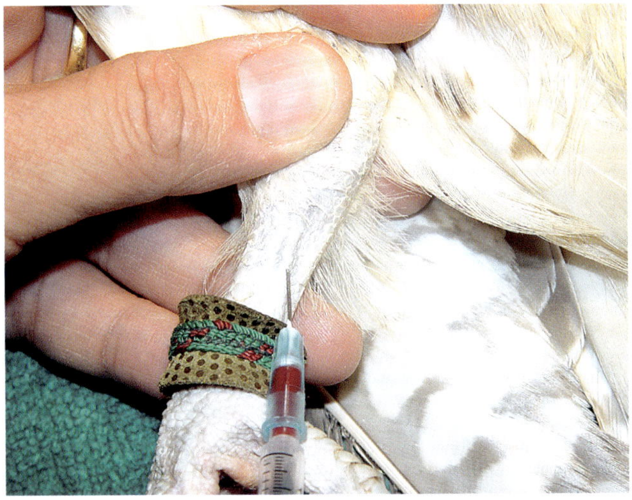

Figure 2.1 c: Blood sampling from a caudal tibial vein (*Vena metatarsalis plantaris superficialis*).

Blood samples should be taken in a quiet and clean environment. Physiological leucocytosis (high white blood cell count) occurs as a result of excitement or stress.

EDTA is a suitable anticoagulant for falcon blood. However, one should be aware that haemolysis occurs when blood from other avian species, such as ostriches, corvids and kookaburras, are mixed with EDTA. For these species, heparin or citrate tubes should be used. Blood should be examined grossly for colour, clots and evidence of erythrocyte agglutination. The presence of lipids may result in a milky red blood sample.

Different blood collection tubes are used for falcon haematology and biochemistry (Table 2.1, Figure 2.2).

Table 2.1: Blood collection tubes for falcons

	Haematology	Biochemistry	Manufacturer
1	Microtainer K_2 EDTA 0.5 ml	–	Becton Dickinson
2	Microtainer EDTA 0.5 ml	–	Teklab Ltd. – U.K.
3	Lithium Heparin 5 ml	–	Becton Dickinson
4	Vacutainer K_3E 4.5 ml	–	Becton Dickinson
5	Vacutainer Lithium Heparin 2 ml	–	Becton Dickinson
6	Lithium Heparin 0.5 ml	–	Teklab Ltd. – U.K.
7	–	Microtainer Tm Brand SST (0.6 ml)	Becton Dickson
8	–	Microtainer Serum Seperator (0.5 ml)	Becton Dickson

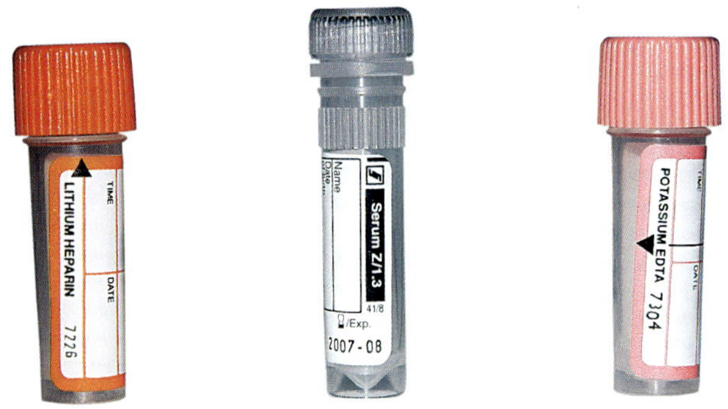

Figure 2.2: Samples of avian blood collection tubes.

There are a number of variables which may affect the results of laboratory tests.

These include:

- Individual variation such as breed, sex, age, fitness
- Sample collection, handling and transportation
- Laboratory equipment and analytical methodology

Automated haematology system

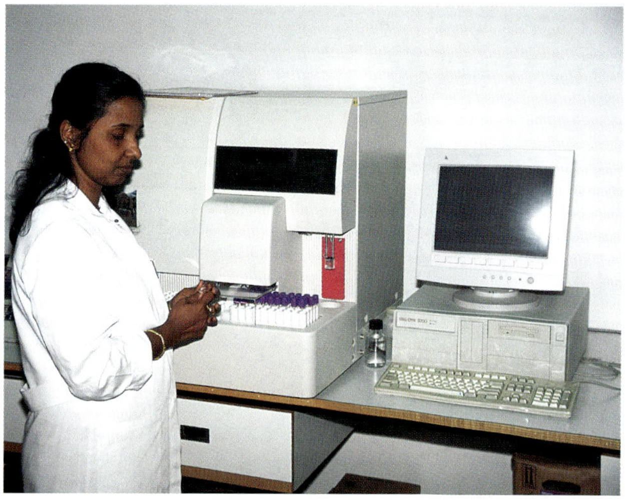

Figure 2.3: Automated haematological analyser.

Complete blood counts (CBC) are commonly performed as part of a presurgical-screen or as part of a »well-animal« care. The availability of semi automated or automated haematology analysers offers veterinary practitioners and animal owners a more efficient and more precise testing system than that achieved using manual methods. To ensure accuracy of results, in-house and external quality control programmes are essential, as unreliable results are misleading and often worse than no results at all.

A wide variety of instruments are available, most of which are specifically designed for human blood analyses. However, more recently, analysers have also become available for nearly all domestic animals in association with multiple pre-programmed settings. Today, advanced haematology systems use flow cytometry to count and identify blood cells in veterinary samples. As cells pass through the laser beam, they absorb and scatter light. Interruptions in the light beam can be used to determine cell counts, whereas changes in light are used to determine cell size and internal complexity or density. For the evaluation of haematology parameters of falcon blood, we used a Cell Dyn 3500 analyser (Abbott Laboratory, North Chicago IL) (Fig. 2.3).

This analyser uses flow cytometry to count and identify blood cells in samples obtained from a variety of animal species. The fully automated instrument measures red blood cell (RBC), white blood cell (WBC) and platelet (thrombocyte; PLT) counts. Gain settings for the laser were modified to allow us to store reference values for a large number of species (camel, goat, sheep, dog, cat, cow, gazelle, horse, avian) and human. Parameters for such species were verified by processing more than 20 blood samples from clinically normal animal species in parallel with manual counts. However, due to the nucleated red blood cells of avians, only RBC, WBC and packed cell volume (PCV; haematocrit) were calculated on this machine. Haemoglobin (HB), mean cellular volume (MCV) and mean cellular haemoglobin (MCH) were calculated using the following formula (Table 2.2).

Table 2.2: Calculation and assessment of red blood cell indices

Erythrocyte Indices	Calculation	Assessment
Haemoglobin HB (g/dl)	$HB = \frac{HCT}{3}$	–
Mean cellular volume MCV (fl)	$MCV = \frac{HCT \times 10}{RBC}$	Differential of erythrocytes into micro, normo and macrocytes
Mean cellular haemoglobin MCH (pg)	$MCH = \frac{HB \times 10}{RBC}$	Differential of hyper and hypochromic anaemia

In birds, the haemoglobin occupies one-third of the red blood cell volume. Therefore an estimation of the haemoglobin concentration can be made by dividing the haematocrit (HCT, PCV) by 3.

WBCs are identified by a Cell Dyn 3500 Analyser with a novel approach referred to as Multi Angle Polarized Scatter Separation (for details see the company's excellent manual). This system works very well with mammalian blood, but cannot be used in avians (Figure 2.4 a, b), for reasons described below.

The below Cell Dyn 3500 haematology reports of a healthy camel (Figure 2.4 a) and a healthy falcon (Figure 2.4 b), illustrates firstly how Multi Angle Polarized Scatter Seperation results in the determination of each of the WBC indices in mammalian blood, and secondly why such a system cannot be used for the analysis of avian blood. The instrument records in graphical display 2 scatter plots and 2 histogrammes. The leukocyte cytogramme on the upper left, separates white blood cells on the basis of size and complexity: Lymphocytes (blue) and basophils (when present) fall into the lowest cluster, with basophils appearing slightly to the right of lymphocytes. Monocytes (purple) appear in a cluster above lymphocytes (blue); neutrophils (red-brown) and eosinophils (green) cluster above and slightly to the right of monocytes (purple). The above right scatter photo separates eosinophils (green) from neutrophils (red).

The lower graphics show histogrammes of RBC (left) and white blood cell impedance count (WIC). In the complexity scatter plot of the falcon sample, cells extend into the lymphocyte area (red cells). In this situation, the instrument shows a NRBC flag, indicating the presence of nucleated RBC and also that it has chosen the WOC count (= optical method). The WIC (= impedance method) count is higher than the WOC count due to the present of NRBC. WIC is not able to discriminate NRBC and is therefore automatically eliminated from the WOC count by a dynamic threshold. The reason for the failure with automated leukocyte determinations in avians, is the similarity between the different leukocytes with respect to size and shape of the cells, the nucleus and the granules and the presence of nucleated RBCs. Furthermore, in falcons the lymphocytes are very similar in size and appearance to thrombocytes and cannot be differentiated electronically.

Consequently, all leukocyte differential counts for falcons were manually performed according to the following pattern (Figure 2.5).

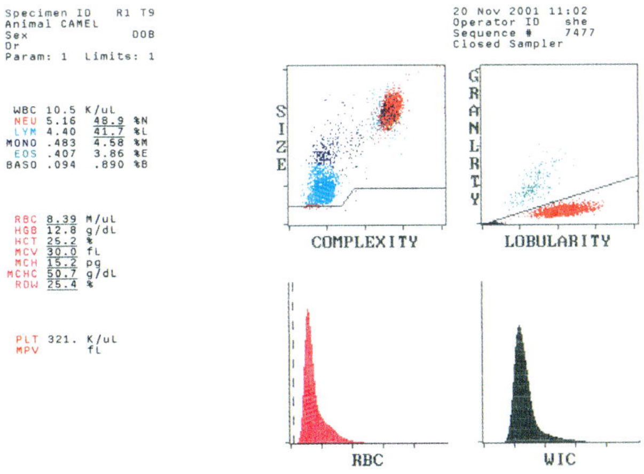

Figure 2.4 a: Haematology report of camel blood.

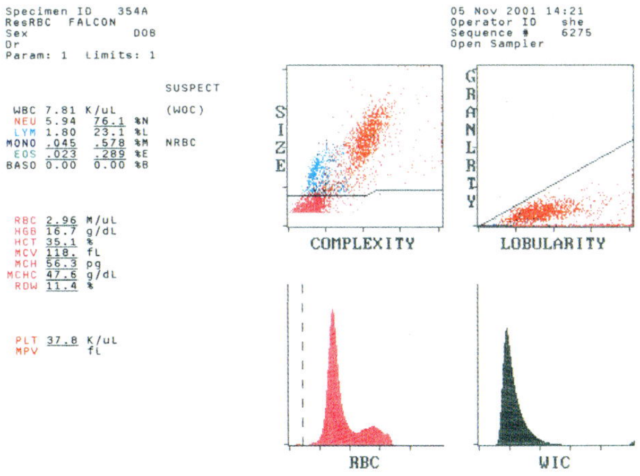

Figure 2.4 b: Haematology report of falcon blood.

Differential WBC counts require the preparation of stained blood smears. The optimal area for evaluation is the front half of the smear behind the feathered edge.

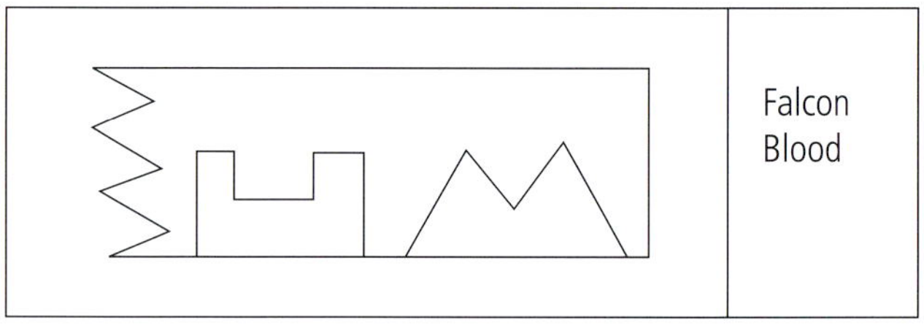

Figure 2.5: Pattern of slide film examination.

Blood film preparation and staining

Blood films should be prepared as soon as possible after blood sample collection to avoid artefactual changes. Blood films are prepared in various ways, including the slide (wedge) method, the cover slip method and the automated slide spinner method. It is essential, that intact cells are present on the slide, enabling accurate examination and differential leucocyte counts to be made.

The importance of producing high quality avian blood smears cannot be over-emphasized. The quality of the final stained smear directly influences the accuracy of the diagnosis. Smears made at the time of blood collection, reflect the morphological changes of blood cells at that point. Prolonged or inappropriate blood storage may have a negative impact on the quality of the cells, and subsequent examination of smears may reveal artefactual cellular changes including vacuolation, swelling and increased numbers of smudge cells. Additionally, contamination of blood smears with dust particles or stain precipitates may result in artefacts, which may be mistaken for bacteria or parasites. It is therefore extremely important, to use clean slides and freshly prepared stains. Blood should only be obtained from live animals, as artefacts, which are caused by disintegrating cells are often found in post mortem blood samples.

A slide stainer cytocentrifuge was used for all falcon blood tested (Figure 2.6).

Before the slides were mounted in a rotating carousel, the slide blood film method was carried out as described below (Figure 2.7).

Once prepared, the slides are immediately dried on a warm air setting (Electrothermal, England, Figure 2.8).

Standard haematology reagents used for the slide stainer cytocentrifuge consist of separate eosin and thiazin (azur B, methylene blue) stains plus a light eosin rinse, all in aqueous solution. Anhydrous methanol is used for fixation. It is a rapid and consistent staining method and stains are exceptionally stable.

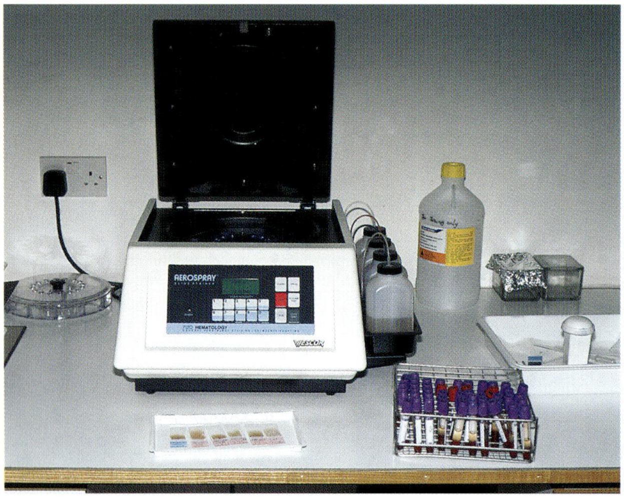

Figure 2.6: Slide stainer cytocentrifuge.

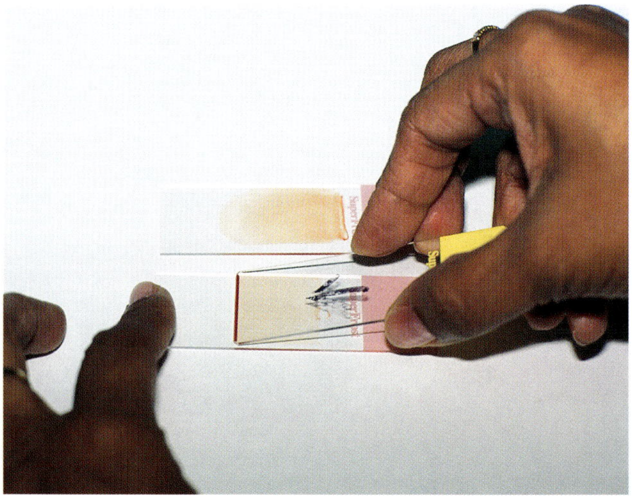

Figure 2.7: A small drop of mixed blood is placed on the end of a clean glass slide and a second glass slide (spreader slide) is placed on the first slide at about 30 degrees angle in front of the drop of blood. The spreader slide is then pushed forward.

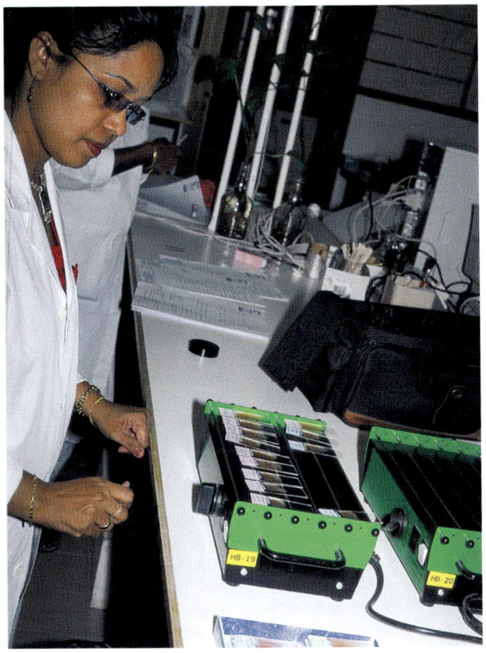

Quantification and examination of the cellular constituents of falcon blood may reveal:

- various types of anaemia with low RBC, HCT (PCV) and HB
- dehydration / haemoconcentration with elevated RBC, HCT and HB
- bacterial infections with elevated WBC count and neutrophilia, lymphocytosis or monocytosis
- viral infections and endo and enterotoxaemias with low WBC count and heteropenia
- parasitic infections or allergies with eosinophilia in some cases

Figure 2.8: Haematology slides drying on a slide dryer.

Reference ranges

It is difficult to define the terminology »normal values« but reference ranges, which are presented on the next pages, relate to data from different clinically normal falcon species. As mentioned earlier, it is sometimes difficult to obtain »normal« values due to changes which may occur during handling stress at the time of venipuncture or following delays in blood analyses.

The references ranges were assumed to include all values within two standard deviations (SD), either side of the mean. The number (n) of falcons tested varied for each species, because firstly the volume of blood sent to the laboratory was often insufficient to conduct all tests offered, and secondly because not all tests were required for each falcon.

Clinicians and clinical pathologists must have some knowledge on which to determine the significance of the results. Textbook references are often not applicable as analytical methodology varies widely between laboratories, and consequently it would be ideal to establish normal parameters for individual birds from the same laboratory over several years or at least over a hunting season to detect early changes. This can be simply achieved by feeding results in a standard database programme.

Haematology values of clinically normal falcons are presented in the following Tables 2.4, 2.5, 2.6, 2.7, 2.8, 2.9, 2.10, 2.11. Due to the high numbers of EDTA blood samples received at CVRL, except for Altai falcons, values of the different falcon species are also presented separately. However, this strategy could not be maintained for the plasma chemistry due to a lower amount of samples received. Values from different falcon species are therefore summarized in Table 2.17, and in Table 2.18 figures are presented from the known literature.

Table 2.3: Explanations of abbreviations for haematology parameters and their SI Units

Abbreviations	Parameters	SI Units
RBC	Red blood cells	$x10^{12}$/l
HB	Haemoglobin	g/dl
HCT	Haematocrit (Packed cell volume = PCV)	l/l
MCV	Mean cellular volume	fl
MCH	Mean cellular haemoglobin	pg
WBC	White blood cells	$x10^{9}$/l
HETERO	Heterophils	%
LYMPHO	Lymphocytes	%
MONO	Monocytes	%
EOS	Eosinophils	%
BASO	Basophils	%

The Système International d'Unites (SI) was recommended for use in the health professions by the World Health Assembly (WHA) in May, 1977. Use of SI is strongly recommended, and many scientific journals now require that units be expressed in SI terms.

2

Table 2.4: Summarized haematology values of 2018 samples from 7 different clinically normal falcon species

Parameters	*Units*	*Mean ± SD*
RBC	x10¹²/l	3.21 ± 0.30
HB	g/dl	14.95 ± 1.39
HCT	l/l	0.45 ± 0.04
MCV	fl	139.85 ± 6.33
MCH	pg	46.42 ± 2.55
WBC	x10⁹/l	9.64 ± 3.96
HETERO	%	59.80 ± 12.87
LYMPHO	%	34.84 ± 12.88
MONO	%	4.46 ± 2.77
EOS	%	0.43
BASO	%	0.16

Table 2.5: Haematology values of 187 clinically normal Gyr falcons

Parameters	*Units*	*Mean ± SD*
RBC	x10¹²/l	3.23 ± 0.28
HB	g/dl	15.00 ± 1.33
HCT	l/l	0.45 ± 0.04
MCV	fl	139.32 ± 5.44
MCH	pg	45.78 ± 1.84
WBC	x10⁹/l	8.71 ± 3.80
HETERO	%	58.53 ± 12.90
LYMPHO	%	37.54 ± 12.98
MONO	%	3.72 ± 2.50
EOS	%	0.20
BASO	%	0.00

Table 2.6: Haematology values of 990 clinically normal Gyr hybrid falcons*

Parameters	*Units*	*Mean ± SD*
RBC	x10¹²/l	3.14 ± 0.31
HB	g/dl	14.67 ± 1.33
HCT	l/l	0.44 ± 0.04
MCV	fl	140.13 ± 8.10
MCH	pg	46.21 ± 2.71
WBC	x10⁹/l	9.43 ± 5.15
HETERO	%	60.42 ± 14.68
LYMPHO	%	34.37 ± 14.23
MONO	%	4.73 ± 3.67
EOS	%	0.31
BASO	%	0.04

* Gyr hybrid = mainly Gyr x Saker or Gyr x Peregrine

Table 2.7: Haematology values of 267 clinically normal Gyr x Peregrine falcons

Parameters	*Units*	*Mean ± SD*
RBC	x10¹²/l	3.35 ± 0.12
HB	g/dl	15.33 ± 0.62
HCT	l/l	0.46 ± 0.02
MCV	fl	137.31 ± 4.15
MCH	pg	45.70 ± 3.43
WBC	x10⁹/l	9.31 ± 3.24
HETERO	%	60.00 ± 10.00
LYMPHO	%	37.43 ± 11.18
MONO	%	2.57 ± 1.23
EOS	%	0.00
BASO	%	0.00

2

Table 2.8: Haematology values of 138 clinically normal Peregrine falcons

Parameters	*Units*	*Mean ± SD*
RBC	$x10^{12}/l$	3.18 ± 0.50
HB	g/dl	14.67 ± 2.06
HCT	l/l	0.44 ± 0.06
MCV	fl	138.43 ± 6.60
MCH	pg	46.13 ± 2.10
WBC	$x10^{9}/l$	9.32 ± 4.69
HETERO	%	60.95 ± 12.01
LYMPHO	%	32.00 ± 11.81
MONO	%	6.23 ± 3.65
EOS	%	0.52
BASO	%	0.26

Table 2.9: Haematology values of 146 clinically normal Saker falcons

Parameters	*Units*	*Mean ± SD*
RBC	$x10^{12}/l$	3.18 ± 0.29
HB	g/dl	15.00 ± 1.46
HCT	l/l	0.45 ± 0.04
MCV	fl	141.50 ± 5.89
MCH	pg	47.17 ± 1.73
WBC	$x10^{9}/l$	10.21 ± 3.53
HETERO	%	61.78 ± 11.16
LYMPHO	%	31.11 ± 11.46
MONO	%	4.72 ± 3.02
EOS	%	1.12
BASO	%	0.40

Table 2.10: Haematology values of 290 clinically normal falcons of unknown species*

Parameters	*Units*	*Mean ± SD*
RBC	$x10^{12}/l$	3.16 ± 0.30
HB	g/dl	15.00 ± 1.54
HCT	l/l	0.45 ± 0.05
MCV	fl	142.40 ± 7.80
MCH	pg	47.46 ± 3.48
WBC	$x10^{9}/l$	10.83 ± 3.34
HETERO	%	57.09 ± 16.50
LYMPHO	%	36.58 ± 15.59
MONO	%	4.79 ± 2.53
EOS	%	0.43
BASO	%	0.23

* species not mentioned on the requisition forms

Table 2.11: Haematology values of 3 clinically normal Altai falcons *

Parameters	*Units*	*Mean ± SD*
RBC	$x10^{12}/l$	3.37 ± 0.38
HB	g/dl	16.33 ± 1.65
HCT	l/l	0.49 ± 0.05
MCV	fl	145.40 ± 3.26
MCH	pg	48.45 ± 0.26
WBC	$x10^{9}/l$	15.07 ± 5.31
HETERO	%	61.33 ± 20.23
LYMPHO	%	27.33 ± 17.93
MONO	%	11.33 ± 2.31 **
EOS	%	0.00
BASO	%	0.00

* excluded from Table 2.4

** these are wild-caught falcons, monocytosis is caused by restraining stress

2

Glossary of terms

Normochromasia:	Normal orange-pink colour of erythrocytes
Polychromasia:	The presence of bluish-red erythrocytes. Polychromatophilic erythrocytes are reticulocytes
Hypochromasia:	Decreased haemoglobin concentration in red blood cells shows increased central pallor
Anisocytosis:	Variation in erythrocyte diameter
Normocytosis:	Presence of normal erythrocytes
Poikilocytosis:	Abnormally shaped erythrocytes
Reticulocytes:	Immature erythrocytes
Polycythaemia:	Increased number of erythrocytes
Karyorrhexis:	Rupture of cell nucleus
Karyolysis:	Dissolution of cell nucleus
Erythropoiesis:	Production of erythrocytes
Erythrocytosis (Polycythaemia):	Increase of erythrocytes

Morphology of normal falcon blood cells

In all vertebrates except mammals, the erythrocytes are oval shaped and nucleated. Erythropoiesis takes place in the bone marrow. Avian erythrocytes are larger than mammalian red blood cells. When cells mature, the size of the nucleus decreases and the volume of cytoplasm increases. The mature erythrocyte has an oval, centrally positioned nucleus. The cytoplasm stains orange-pink. Active erythropoiesis in birds is based on the number of polychromatic cells and on the appearance and size of the nucleus and cytoplasm in blood films, and not on reticular material. Reticular material is virtually present in all erythrocytes of birds and therefore makes interpretation very difficult. The degree of erythrocyte polychromasia is an indication of erythrogenesis, and peripheral blood films from clinically normal birds show a 1–5 % erythrocyte polychromasia. Other evidence of active erythropoiesis is the presence of bi-nucleated immature erythrocytes and an increase in the number of normal immature erythrocytes in the peripheral blood. However, in cases of non-anaemic falcons, these cells indicate abnormal erythropoiesis. Immature erythrocytes may also indicate abnormal erythropoiesis or an early release from the haematopoietic tissue following anoxic insult or toxicity.

Erythrocytes, heterophils and monocytes are not difficult to identify in avian blood films. In birds, the cells analogous with mammalian neutrophils are known as heterophils. They possess brick-red, cigar-shaped granules.

Extensive experience is required in the identification of lymphocytes and thrombocytes. This is especially true in relation to activated thrombocytes, termed megathrombocytes. Thrombocytes may also be confused with disrupted erythrocyte nuclei. Therefore, special attention has been drawn to this general problem in falcons. Thrombocytes of birds are nucleated and significantly larger than mammalian platelets. Normal thrombocytes may be oval, round or spindle-shaped with clear or pale bluish cytoplasm. The nuclear chromatin is dense and clumped. Produced from mononuclear precursors in the bone marrow, thrombocytes are haemostatic blood elements which may also have a phagocytic function. Thrombocytosis occurs in response to haemorrhage or bacterial infection whereas thrombocytopenia is often associated with severe septicaemias and toxaemias. The normal thrombocyte count for falcons is 20,000–30,000/µl blood. Pictures shown on the following pages explain the differences between thrombocytes, lymphocytes and disrupted erythrocyte nuclei.

Eosinophils and basophils are quite rare in avians, and are not easy to detect. Pictures show the distinct morphology of both types of cells. Sometimes it can also be difficult to distinguish between eosinophils and heterophils, especially when heterophils exhibit toxic granulation. However, in healthy birds the heterophils' granules are brick-red and cigar-shaped, whereas in eosinophils they are purple and round. Little is known about the function of eosinophils and basophils. Even in falcons with heavy parasitic burden, we have failed to observe eosinophilias.

Avian basophils are smaller than heterophils and eosinophils and usually display round dark granules in their cytoplasm. Heterophils and eosinophils have a lobed, usually bi-lobed nucleus, whereas basophils have a single round, centrally located nucleus. The nucleus is often hidden by the cytoplasmic granules.

Lymphopoiesis takes place in the bursa of Fabricius in birds and lymphocytes are involved in immunological reactions. An increase in lymphocytes occurs in viral infections and lymphoproliferative disorders. Lymphocytes are divided into 2 functional groups: T-lymphocytes which are responsible for cell-mediated immunity and B-lymphocytes which produce immunoglobulins. Lymphocytes can also be classified into 3 groups according to cell size (small, medium and large). Most normal lymphocytes in the peripheral blood are small and medium, with a round and centrally located nucleus. The amount of cytoplasm varies from a narrow band surrounding the nucleus in small lymphocytes to a wider band in medium and large lymphocytes. The cytoplasm is homogenous and basophilic.

Monocytes are the largest circulating blood cells. They possess a kidney bean-shaped large nucleus and abundant bluish cytoplasm. Their main function is phagocytosis of invading microorganisms, cell debris and necrotic cells. Monocytosis may occur with bacterial, viral, fungal and protozoal disease. Levels above 7 % suggest chronic infection in hunting falcons which warrants a complete check-up. However, higher levels have been observed in clinically normal wild falcons (Table 2.11).

Most of the following haematology and some of the histology figures have been highlighted by red or blue squares in order to focus the readers' attention.

2

The different anaemias in birds

Haemorrhagic anaemia

Blood loss through trauma, blood-sucking insects, coagulopathies, gastrointestinal parasites, ulcers, rupture of internal organs, viral diseases

- regenerative response is common with polychromasia, macrocytosis and anisocytosis

Haemolytic anaemia

Increased destruction of red blood cells through blood parasites like *Plasmodium*, *Aegyptianella*, *Leucocytozoon* and *Babesia* and salmonellosis, enterotoxaemias like clostridiosis, lead toxicosis

- regenerative response is common

Depression anaemia

Decreased erythropoiesis caused by inflammatory diseases like aspergillosis, tuberculosis, chlamydophilosis, and lead intoxication, liver diseases, neoplasia, chemicals

- non-regenerative response with normocytosis and normochromasia

HCT (PCV) and total protein (TP) values are useful indicators for determining the underlying cause of an anaemia (Table 2.12).

Table 2.12: Assessment of HCT and TP

	Elevated TP	Normal TP	Low TP
Low HCT	Depression anaemia non-regenerative	Haemolytic anaemia, regenerative	Haemorrhagic anaemia, blood loss, haemorrhage, regenerative
Normal HCT	Anaemia and dehydration	–	Hypoproteinaemia
Elevated HCT	Dehydration	Polycythaemia	Hypoproteinaemia

2

Avian erythrocytes function similarly to mammalian erythrocytes. Common artefactual abnormalities in erythrocyte morphology include cytoplasmic refractile vacuoles, smudge cell nuclei, and various morphologies induced by stretching cells while preparing the smear.

Microhaematocrit centrifugation is used to determine the packed cell volume (PCV). This method is commonly used to estimate the red cell mass. The haematocrit (HCT) is calculated from measured mean cellular volume and RBC when derived by automated cell counters. Theoretically, the calculated HCT is more accurate than the PCV, but there are no controlled studies to confirm this in avian species.

HCT values less than 0.35 l/l are an indication of anaemia and HCT greater than 0.55 l/l indicate dehydration or erythrocytosis (polycythaemia). Erythrocytosis can be differentiated by total protein (TP): elevated TP indicates dehydration, while normal or low TP levels support erythrocytosis. New falcons which have not been used for falconry have high HCT levels with values around 0.50–0.55 l/l, which drop during training. Many falcons which moult in the U.A.E. suffer from anaemia, which resolves with training. This may take more than a month. Sick falcons with low HCT of 0.25–0.35 l/l require rest and supportive therapy, and HCT values of 0.20–0.15 l/l require blood transfusions.

CVRL does not measure haemoglobin independently, because there is no reliable haemoglobinometer for avians available. Therefore, values are directly linked to HCT. HB values below 13.0 g/dl require therapy.

Pictures of normal haematology of different falcon species

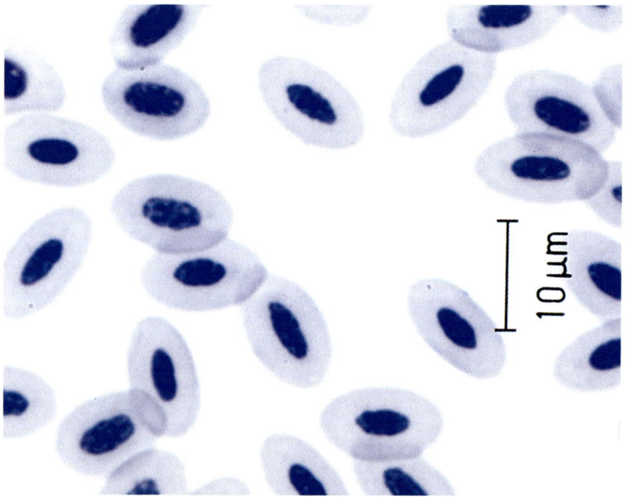

Figure 2.9: Normal red blood cells of a Saker falcon (*Falco cherrug*). Avian erythrocytes are larger than those of most mammals. Their size is directly related to body size (MCV 139.85 ± 6.33 fl).

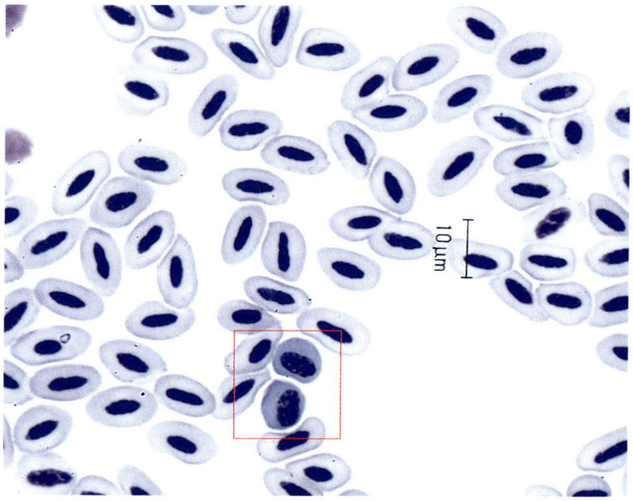

Figure 2.10: Normal blood picture of a clinically normal Peregrine falcon (*Falco peregrinus*) with two immature basophilic erythrocytes.

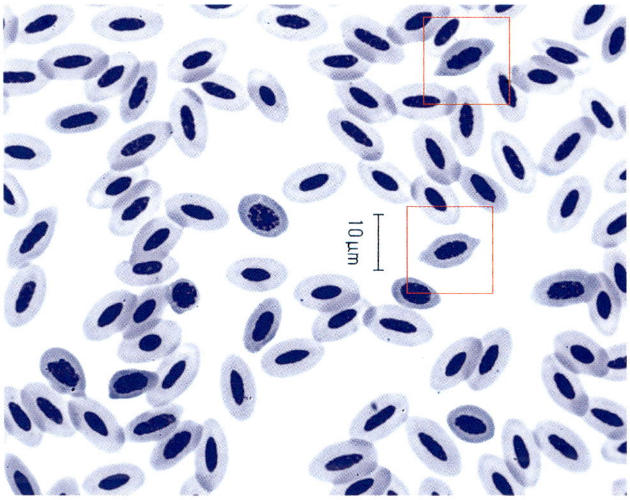

Figure 2.11: Several basophilic erythroblasts; a sign of active erythropoiesis. When cells mature, the amount of cytoplasm increases and the size of the nucleus decreases. Two spindle-shaped cells are also present (highlighted). Blood smear of a Saker falcon.

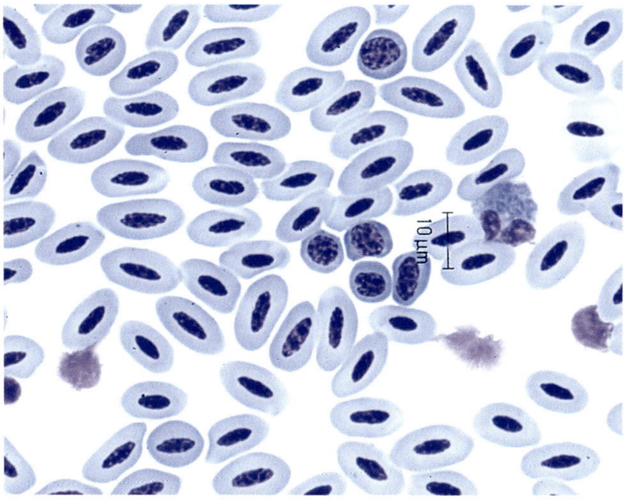

Figure 2.12: Several immature erythrocytes of a Lanner falcon (*Falco biarmicus*).

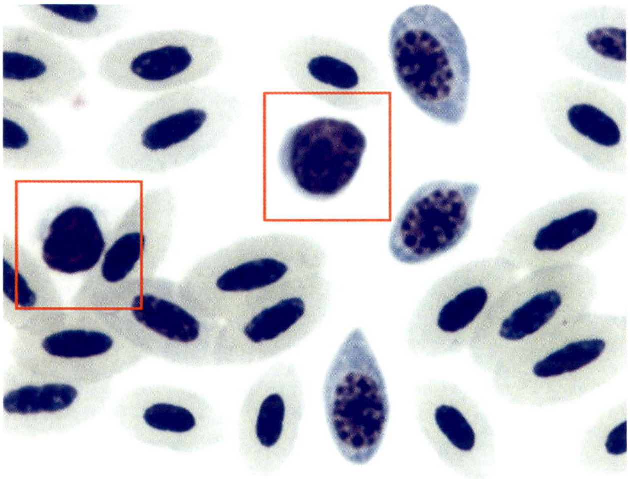

Figure 2.13: Three polychromatic erythroblasts and two thrombocytes in a blood smear of a Peregrine falcon (highlighted) (*Falco peregrinus*).

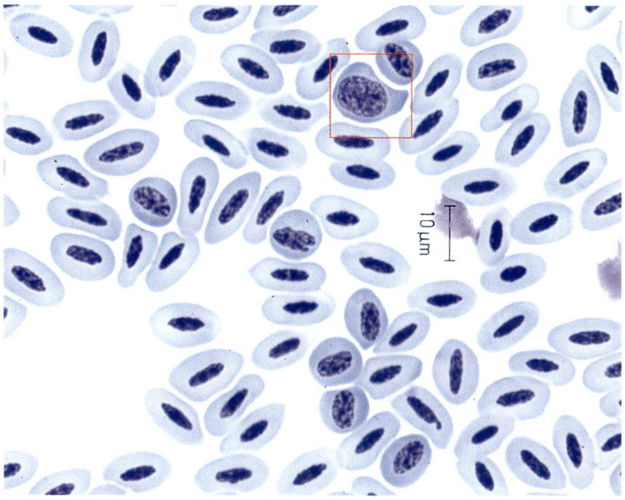

Figure 2.14: Active erythropoiesis with several immature erythrocytes and one erythroblast (highlighted). Regenerative anaemia is often found in young falcons and usually resolves without treatment.

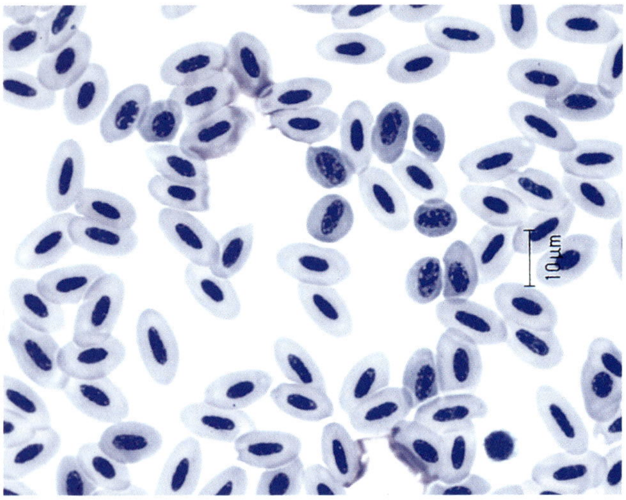

Figure 2.15: Polychromasia: Ten basophilic erythroblasts are visible in the blood smear of a Gyr falcon.

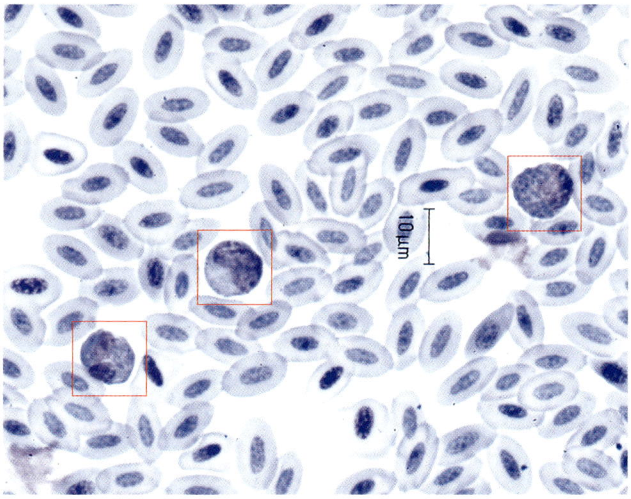

Figure 2.16: Two normal heterophils and one normal monocyte of a Peregrine falcon. The cytoplasmic granules of heterophils are cigar-shaped. These cells are the most common leukocytes seen in avian blood smears.

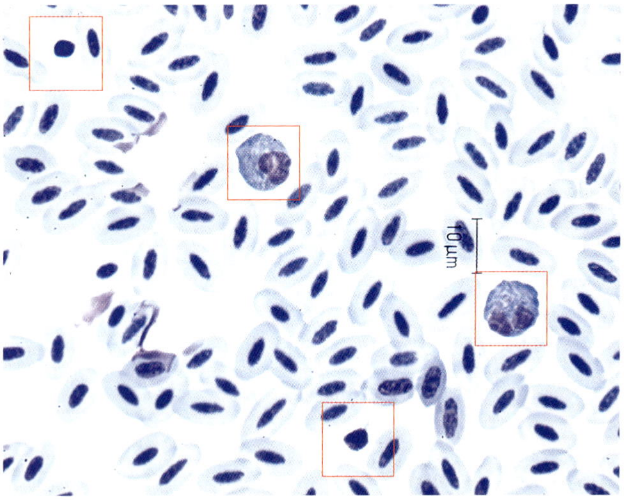

Figure 2.17: Two normal heterophils with distinct granules and two thrombocytes of a clinically normal Gyr x Peregrine hybrid.

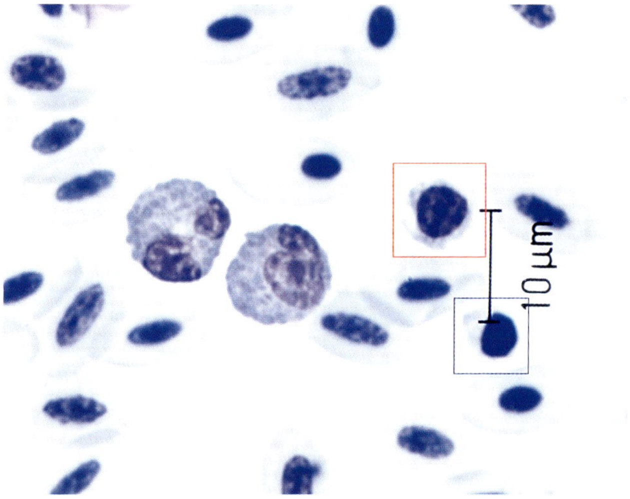

Figure 2.18: Two heterophils of a Saker falcon. The nucleus of both is bi-lobed. One thrombocyte (highlighted in blue) and one lymphocyte are also visible.

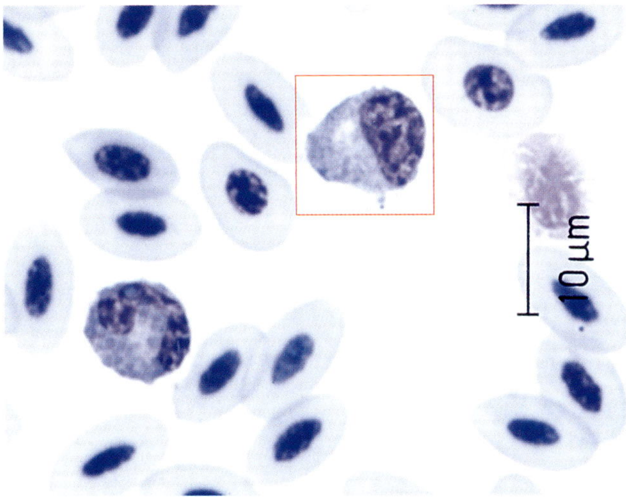

Figure 2.19: One heterophil with a bi-lobed nucleus and one monocyte (highlighted) of a Gyr falcon.

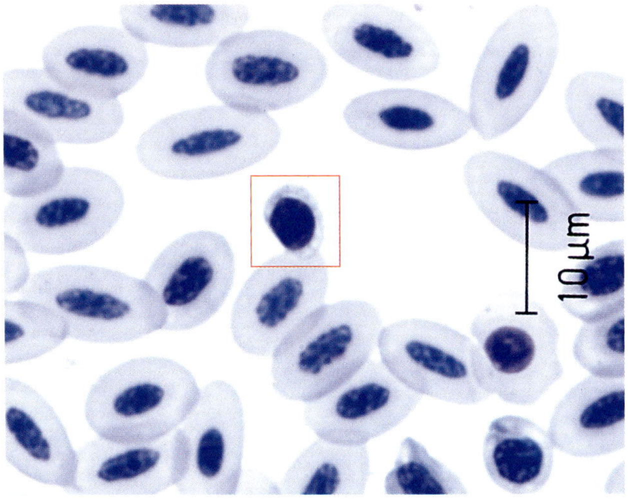

Figure 2.20: One normal thrombocyte of a Peregrine falcon. In avians thrombocytes are surrounded by a pale bluish cytoplasm and possess very condensed nuclei.

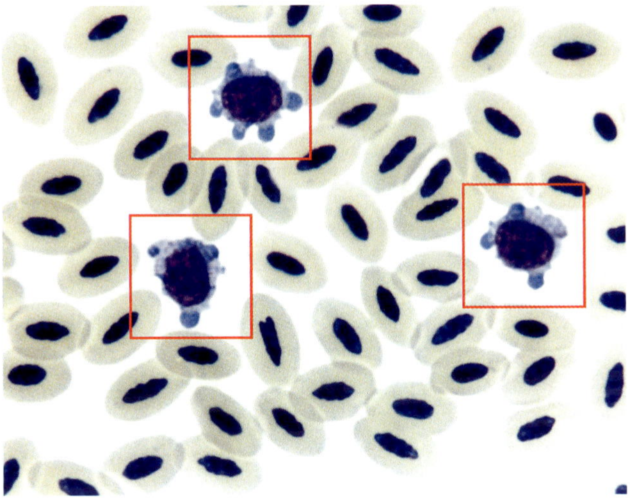

Figure 2.21 a: Three mega thrombocytes of a clinically normal Gyr falcon (*Falco rusticolus*).

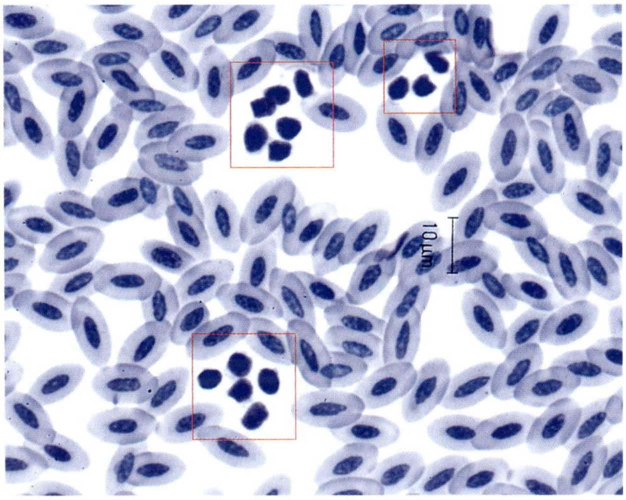

Figure 2.21 b: Three aggregations of thrombocytes.

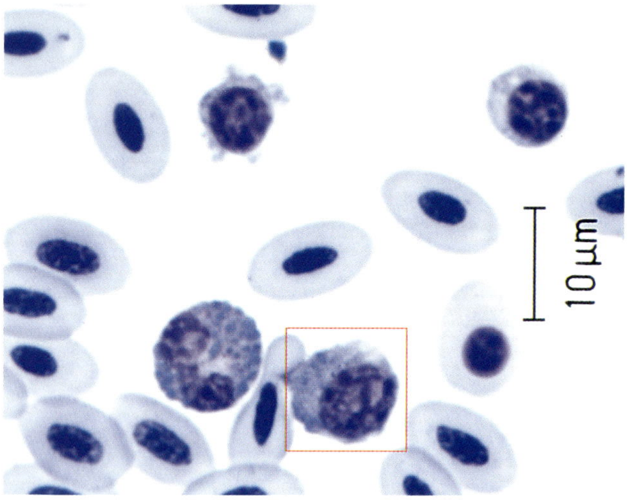

Figure 2.22: Two mega thrombocytes, one heterophil and one reactive lymphocyte (highlighted) of a Gyr hybrid.

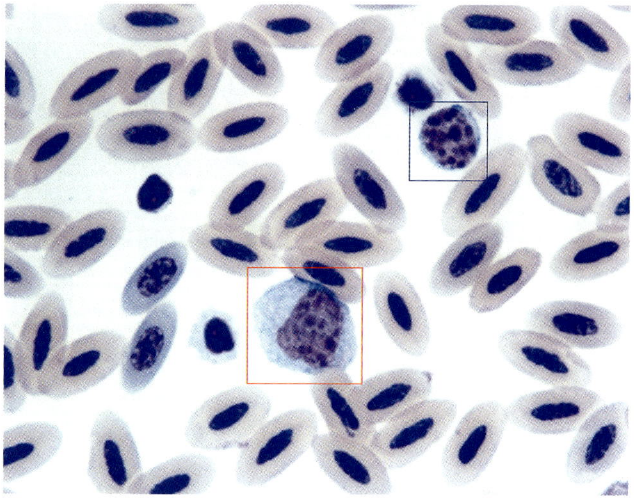

Figure 2.23: One normal monocyte (highlighted in red), one normal lymphocyte (highlighted in blue) and three normal thrombocytes of a clinically normal Gyr hybrid. In avian species, the monocyte is characterized by its large size. The nucleus is commonly »D« or kidney bean shaped.

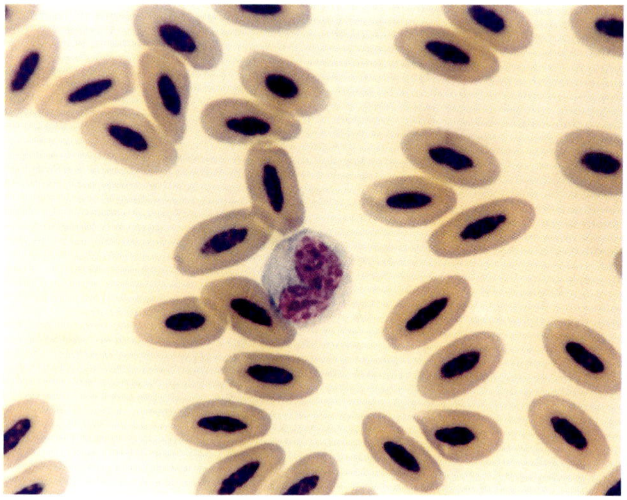

Figure 2.24: One normal monocyte of a Saker falcon (*Falco cherrug*).

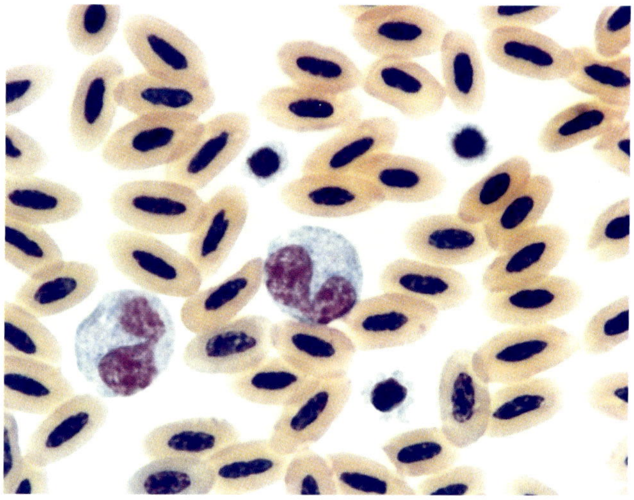

Figure 2.25: Two normal monocytes and three normal thrombocytes of a Peregrine falcon (*Falco peregrinus*). Monocytes do not possess granules.

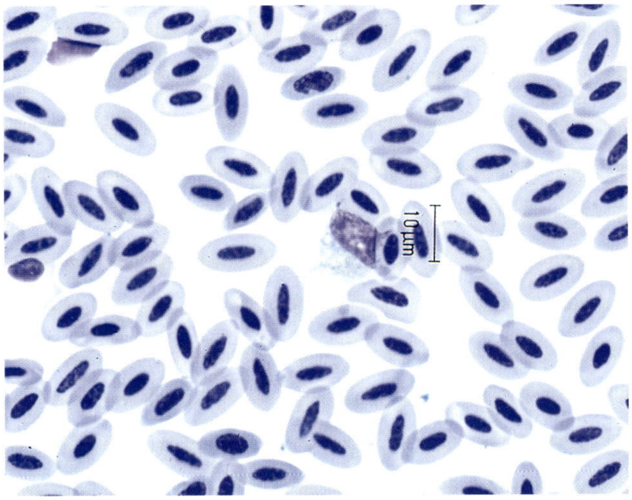

Figure 2.26: A »squeezed« monocyte of a Gyr hybrid.

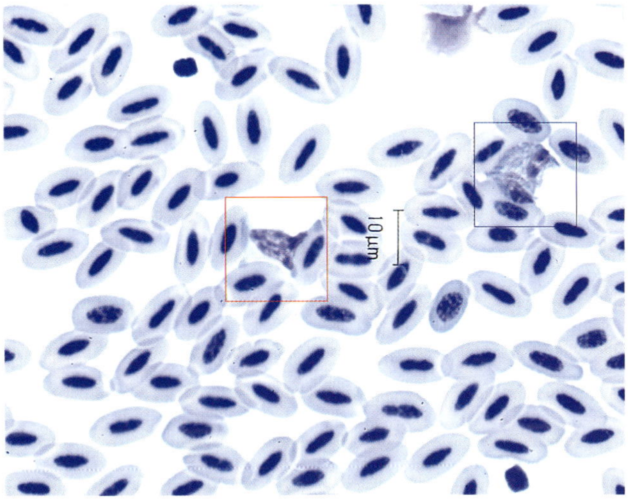

Figure 2.27: One normal lymphocyte (highlighted in red), two thrombocytes and a disrupted heterophil (highlighted in blue) of a Gyr falcon. Lymphocytes in blood smear preparations from birds are frequently found positioned between two erythrocytes.

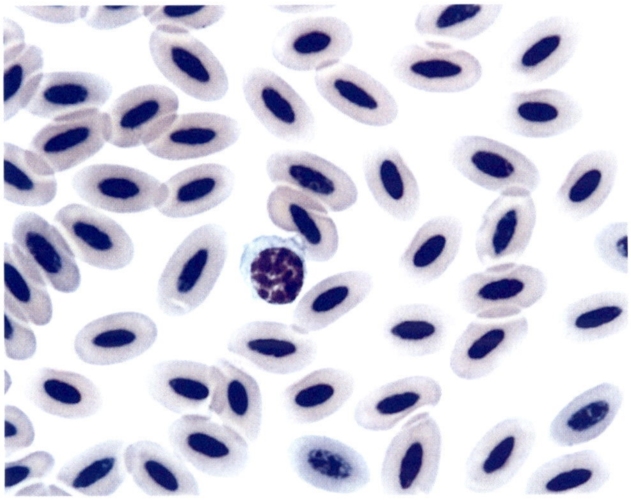

Figure 2.28: A normal lymphocyte of a Peregrine falcon (*Falco peregrinus*).

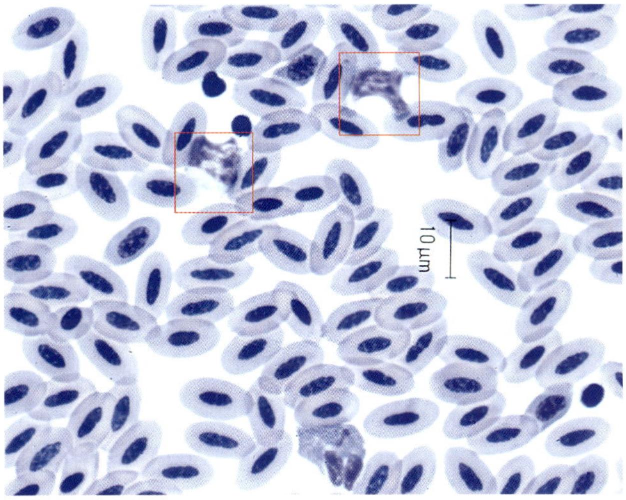

Figure 2.29: Two lymphocytes (highlighted) (squeezed between erythrocytes), one heterophil and three thrombocytes of a clinically normal Gyr hybrid.

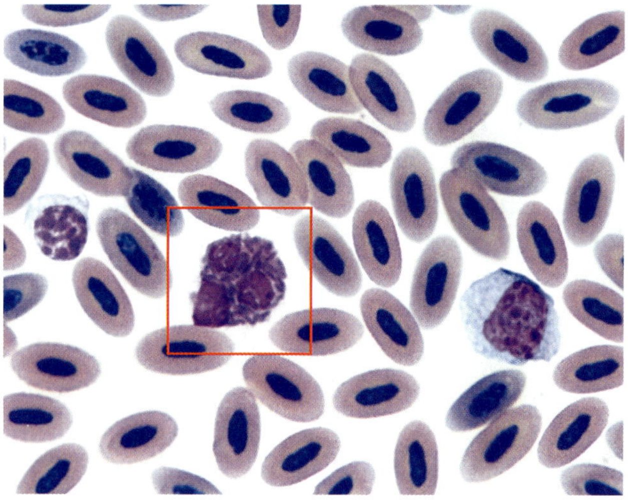

Figure 2.30: One three-lobed heterophil (highlighted), one monocyte and one lymphocyte of a clinically normal Gyr hybrid.

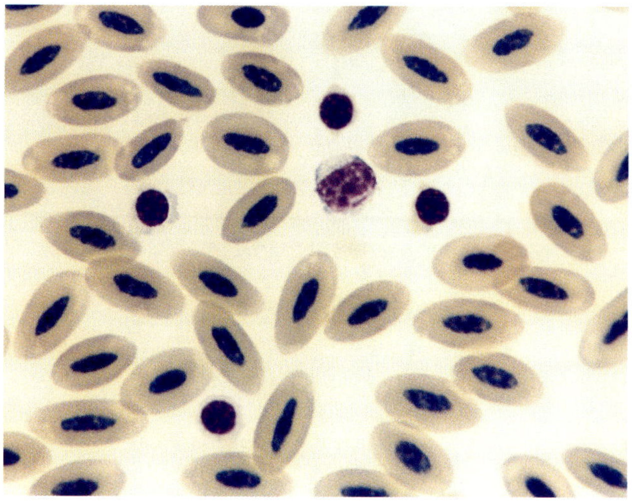

Figure 2.31: A medium sized lymphocyte and four thrombocytes of a Gyr hybrid.

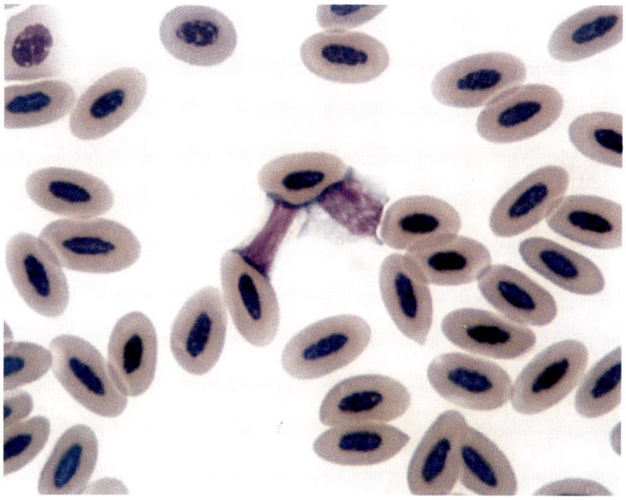

Figure 2.32 a: Two normal lymphocytes of a clinically normal Gyr hybrid.

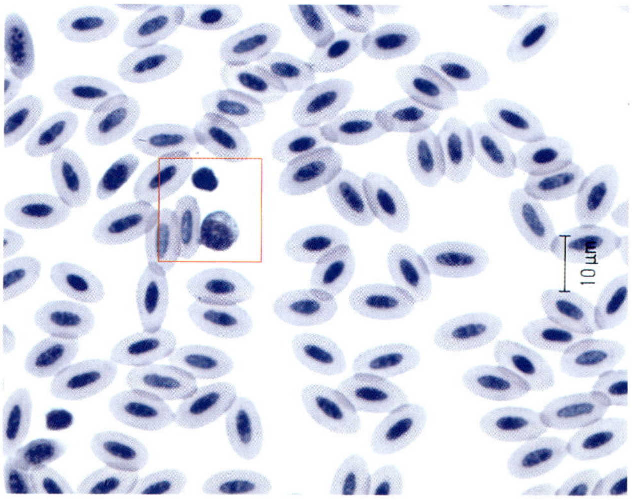

Figure 2.32 b: A lymphocyte positioned adjacent to one (highlighted) of the two thrombocytes of a clinically normal Gyr hybrid.

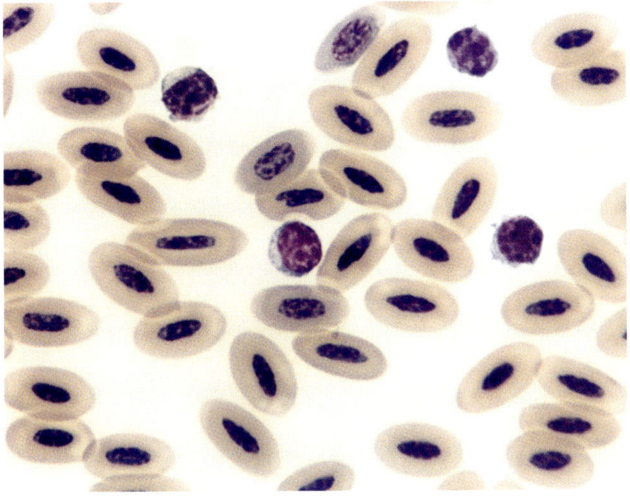

Figure 2.33: Four medium sized lymphocytes of a clinically normal Saker falcon (*Falco cherrug*).

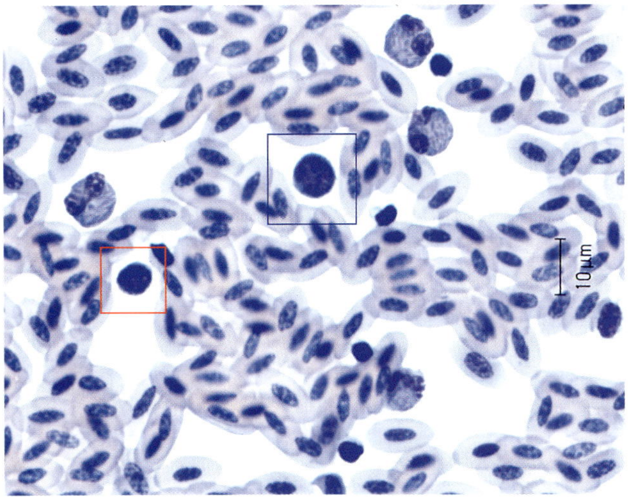

Figure 2.34: Four heterophils, one small lymphocyte (highlighted in red), one medium-sized lymphocyte (highlighted in blue) and six thrombocytes of a Saker falcon; the thrombocyte next to the bar is a mega thrombocyte.

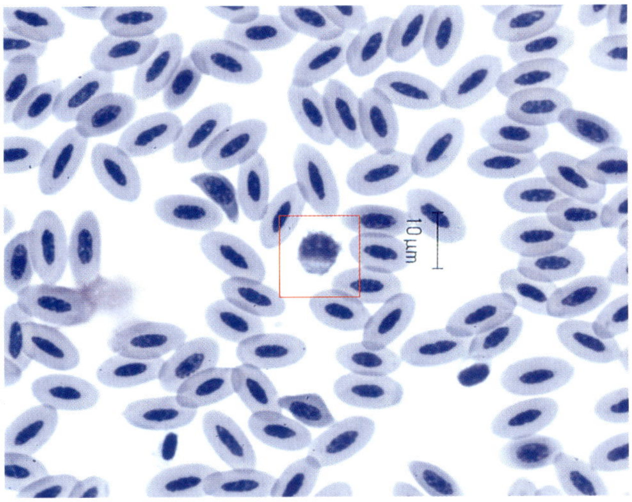

Figure 2.35: Most probably a lymphocyte (highlighted), two thromboyctes and a sickle-shaped erythrocyte of a clinically normal Saker falcon.

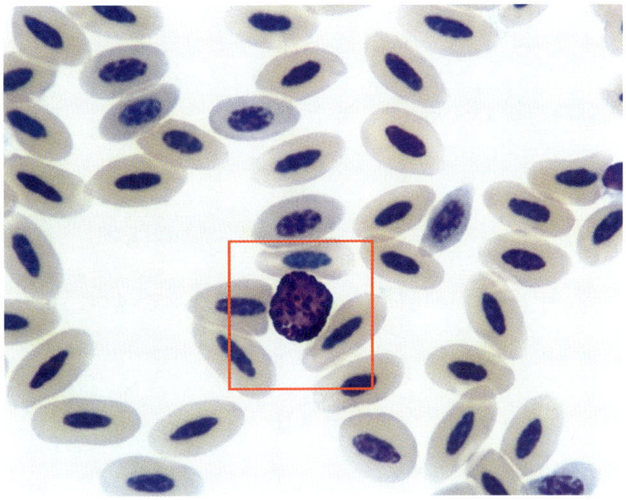

Figure 2.36: A basophil of a clinically normal Saker falcon (*Falco cherrug*).

2

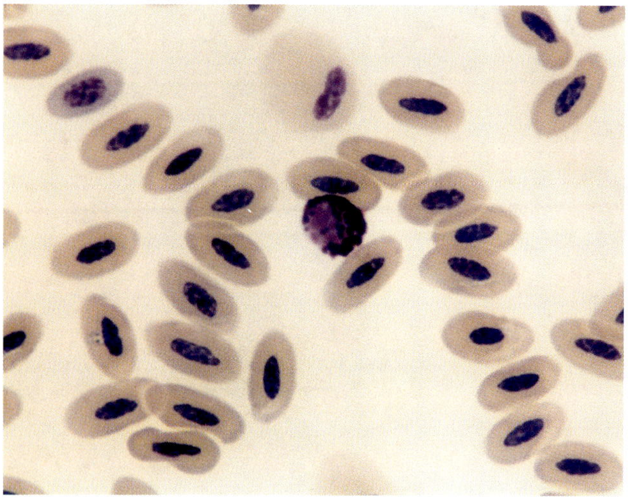

Figure 2.37 a: A basophil of a clinically normal Peregrine falcon (*Falco peregrinus*).

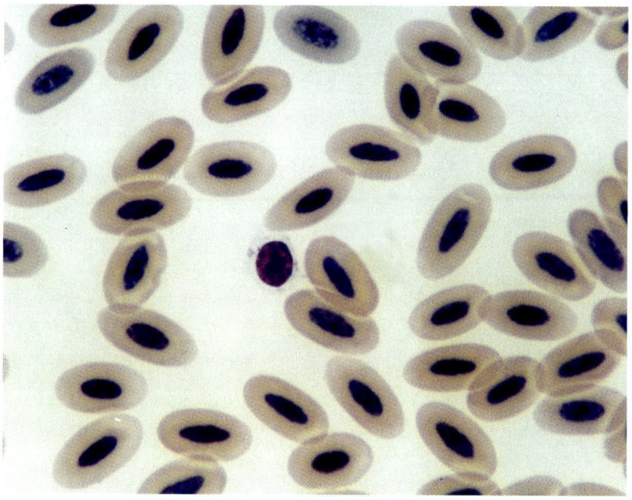

Figure 2.37 b: A thrombocyte of a clinically normal Peregrine falcon (*Falco peregrinus*).

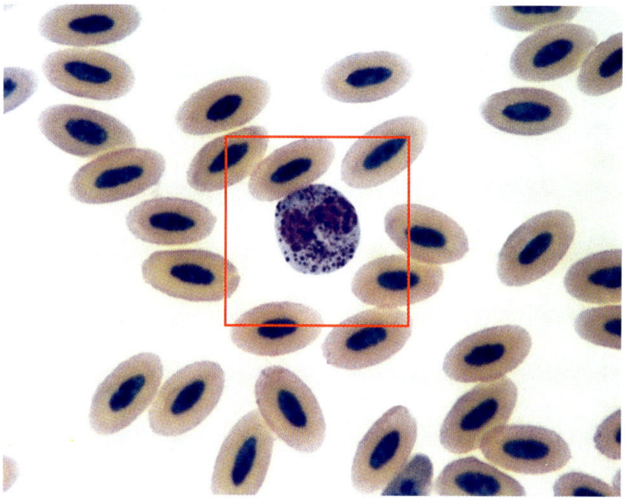

Figure 2.38: An eosinophil of a Gyr hybrid.

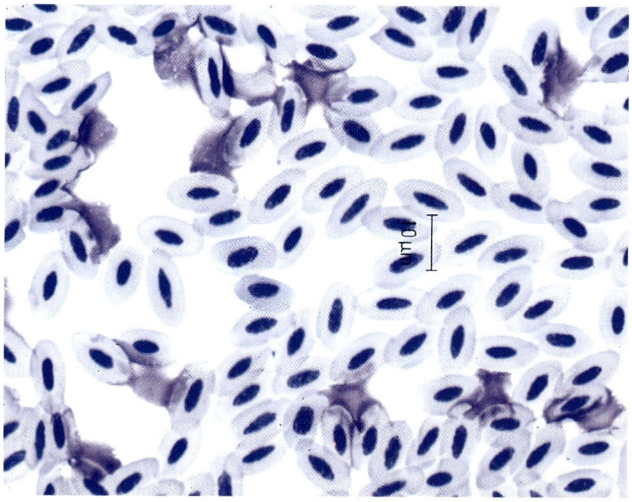

Figure 2.39: This picture shows many smudge cell nuclei in a blood film from a clinically normal Gyr falcon. Count is not possible. The occurrence of smudge cell nuclei indicates that the blood sample is either old or the blood cells have been disrupted during preparation of the smear.

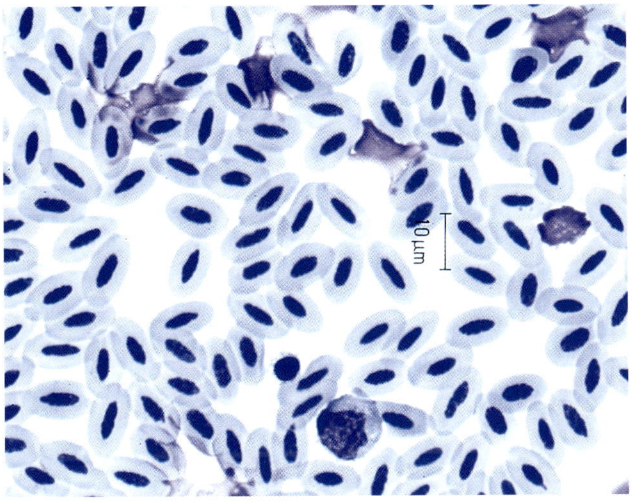

Figure 2.40: One monocyte, one thrombocyte and seven smudge cell nuclei of a Saker falcon. In this case, the staining would require to be repeated or performed on a fresh sample, using fresh stains.

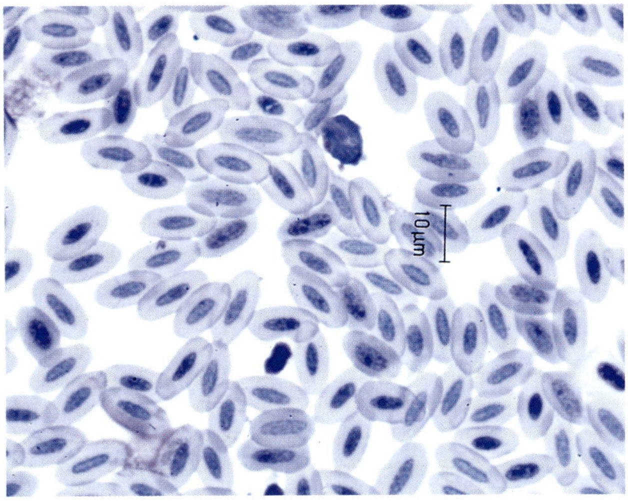

Figure 2.41: Poor staining quality of a blood smear from a Saker falcon. The morphology of the cells is not recognizable. Staining would have to be repeated.

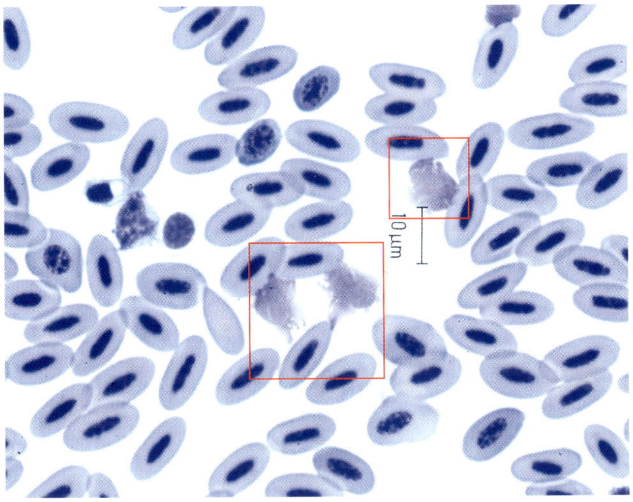

Figure 2.42: Amorphous nuclear material from disrupted erythrocytes. Disruption of a small number of erythrocytes commonly occurs when preparing blood films of avians. Misidentification should be avoided with thrombocytes and lymphocytes. Three immature red cells and one erythroplastiv are also seen.

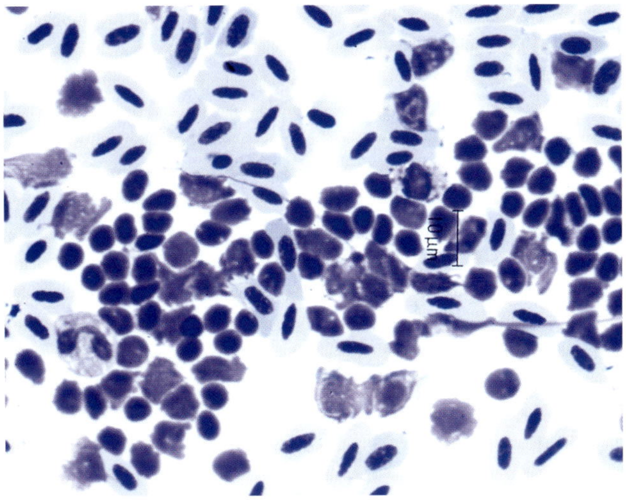

Figure 2.43: Poor preparation of a blood smear from a Gyr x Peregrine hybrid. The morphology of most of the cells is not recognizable.

2

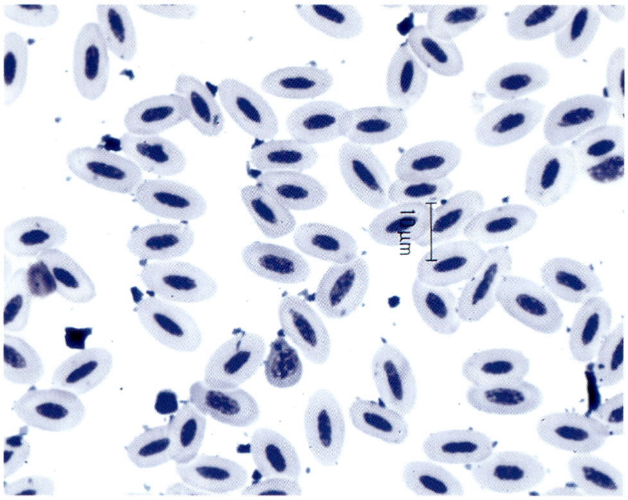

Figure 2.44: Stain precipitates in a stained falcon blood smear indicating the use of old staining solutions or preparation made from powder, which was not adequately filtered.

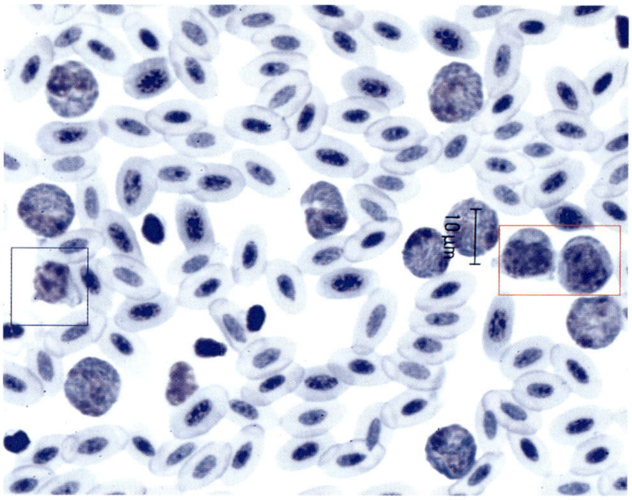

Figure 2.45: Poor staining of a Saker falcon blood. The colour is too light. However, nine heterophils, five thrombocytes and two monocytes (highlighted in red) and one lymphocyte (highlighted in blue) are visible.

Abnormalities in falcon leukocytes

The next section, and the following disease chapters include pictures of various leukocyte abnormalities which may be seen on stained falcon blood smears. Descriptions of these changes are presented here.

Toxic changes in heterophils

Toxic changes in heterophils may occur in viral, bacterial, fungal and metabolic disorders and are associated with systemic illness. They are also observed in intoxications and toxaemias.

Toxic changes are indicated by:

- degranulation and/or variation in size and shape of the granules
- cytoplasmic basophilia
- vacuolisation
- nuclear degeneration

These changes may be reported on a scale from +1 toxicity to +4 toxicity. A +4 score would be associated with:

- marked degranulation, round granules with central bodies
- deep cytoplasmic basophilia
- cytoplasmic vacuolation
- karyorrhexis and/or karyolysis

If less than 25 % of heterophils are affected by toxic changes, this would suggest an early stage of the disorder. Falcons showing +4 score in most of the heterophils in the blood film often have a grave prognosis.

Abnormal lymphocytes

Lymphocyte abnormalities are associated with inflammatory diseases when antigenic stimulation is present. These diseases include aspergillosis, chlamydophilosis, salmonellosis as well as viral diseases like Paramyxovirus-1 infection and herpesvirus infection. The main lymphocyte abnormalities seen are:

- reactive lymphocytes: increased cell size, deep basophilic cytoplasm and reddish nucleus. These lymphocytes produce immunoglobulins and lymphokines (immune response)
- lymphocytes with azurophilic granules (magenta) in their cytoplasm indicate immaturity or toxicity
- lymphocytes with scalloped cytoplasmic borders: a few of these cells may be seen in blood smears of clinically normal falcons, however if increased numbers are observed with marked lymphocytosis, this could be evidence for neoplasia

Appearance of unusual cells

Occasionally unusual cells may appear in the peripheral blood of falcons. They include plasma cells and cells with large round cytoplasmic granules which are colourless. These changes are regarded as artefacts rather than abnormal cells.

Falcon leukogramme

Blood parameters obtained from diseased falcons must differ greatly from normal reference values in order to be considered significant. It would be ideal to receive repeated serial samples from the same falcon to evaluate changes in the leukogramme. One should keep in mind that a »handling leukocytosis« may elevate leukocyte levels above 12,000 to 13,000/µl blood. In general, falcons do not respond to infectious diseases with a high peripheral blood white cell count like mammals and other avian species. They rarely exhibit a total white cell count of more than 15,000 to 17,000/µl blood. Even in advanced aspergillosis, chlamydophilosis or amyloidosis, cases can stabilize and may show reasonable blood pictures.

Leucocytosis

Leucocytosis is the increase in the concentration of heterophils and lymphocytes. It can be caused by handling, inflammation, toxicities, neoplasm, leukaemia. Heterophilia is the increase of heterophils caused by inflammation in association with *Chlamydophila, Mycobacterium, Aspergillus.* Toxic heterophilia occurs with severe systemic illness, such as septicaemia, viraemia, chlamydophilosis, mycotic infections and severe tissue necroses. The degree of heterophil toxicity usually indicates the severity of the falcons' condition.

Leukopenia

Leukopenia is the decrease in the concentration of heterophils and lymphocytes. It is associated with either consumption of the peripheral leukocytes or decreased production. Severe bacterial infections like clostridiosis or certain viral diseases like herpesvirus may cause leukopenia.

Haematological pictures of abnormal leukocytes

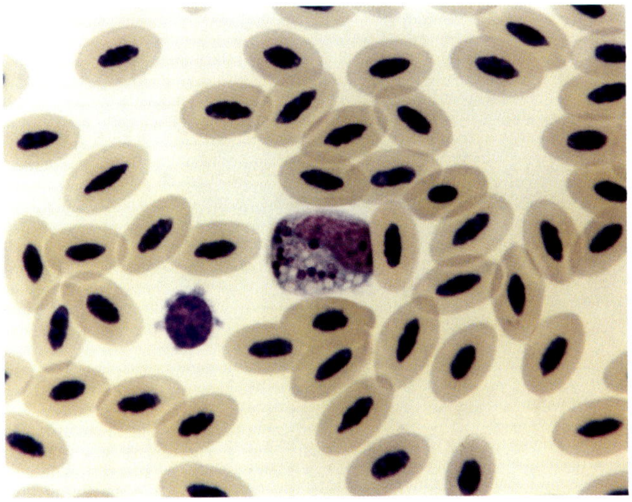

Figure 2.46: A toxic heterophil and a mega thrombocyte of a Peregrine falcon (*Falco peregrinus*). Mild degranulation and loss of lobulation (left shift) in the nucleus (+1).

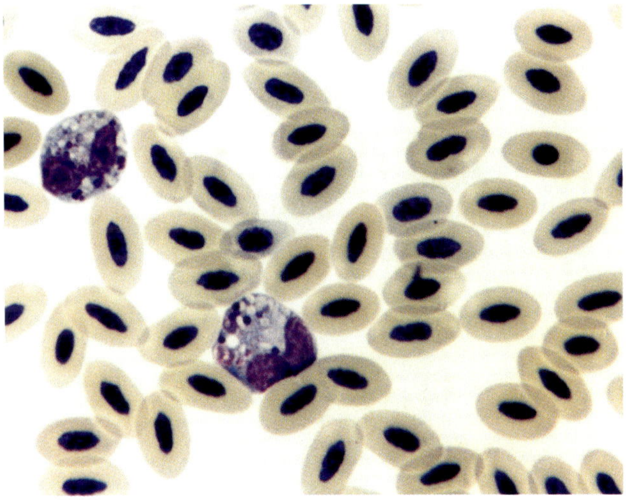

Figure 2.47: Severe toxic changes (+4) of two heterophils of a Gyr falcon (*Falco rusticolus*). The granules are round and basophilic.

2

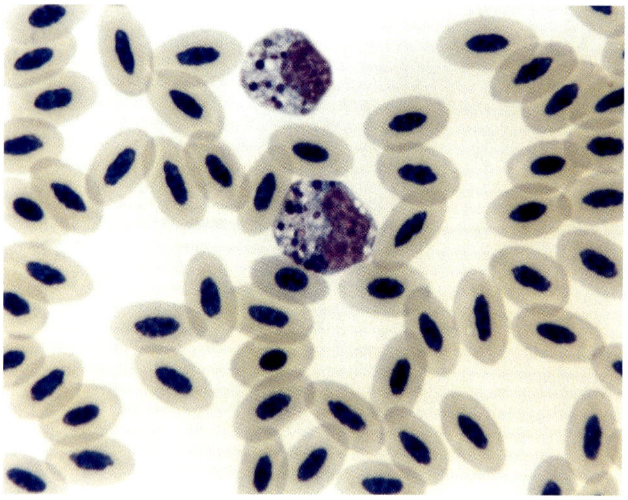

Figure 2.48: Two heterophils with severe toxic changes (+4) of a Saker falcon (*Falco cherrug*). Loss of granulation, left shifted (loss of lobulation) nucleus and large round nucleus stained dark purple in colour.

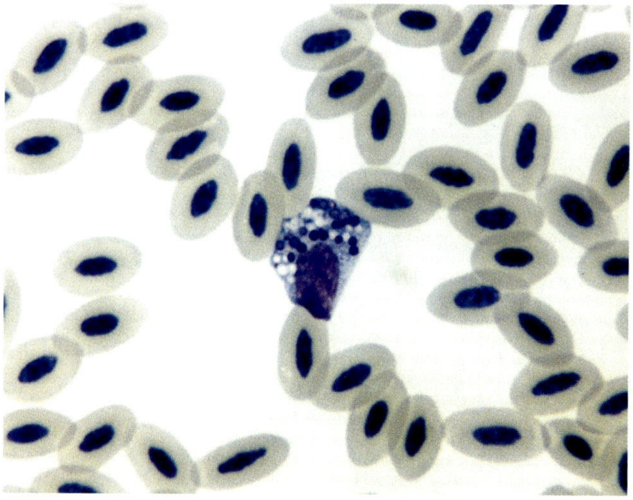

Figure 2.49: One heterophil with severe toxic changes (+4) of a Peregrine falcon (*Falco peregrinus*). Loss of granulation, left shifted (loss of lobulation) nucleus and large round nucleus stained dark purple in colour.

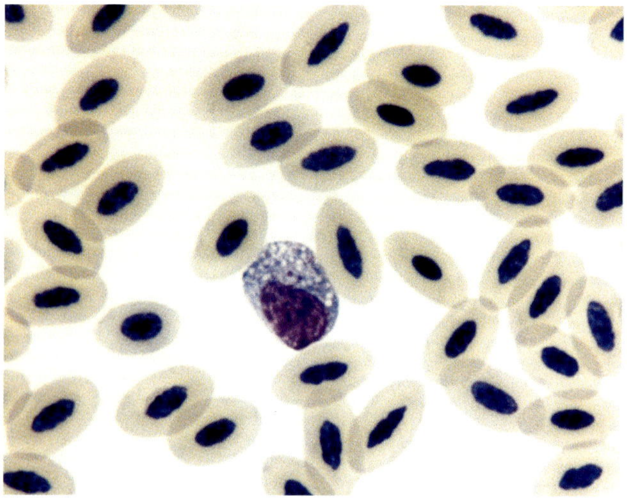

Figure 2.50: One heterophil with complete loss of granulation and left shift (loss of lobulation) of a Gyr hybrid.

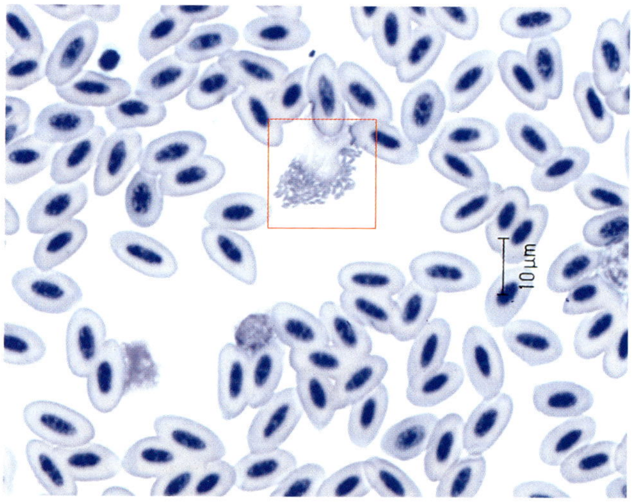

Figure 2.51: A disrupted heterophil from a Peregrine falcon. The cigar-shaped granules are clearly visible.

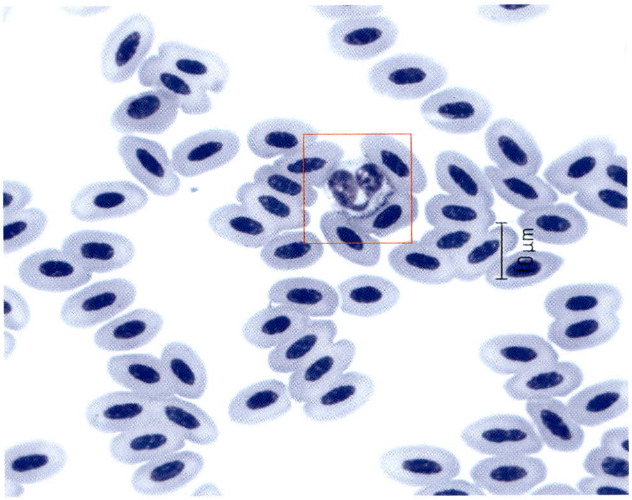

Figure 2.52: A squeezed eosinophil from a Gyr hybrid. The nucleus is bi-lobed, and tiny bluish granules are visible in the cytoplasm.

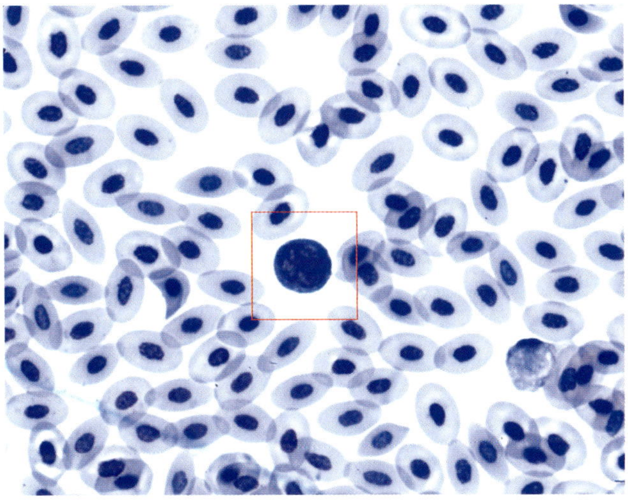

Figure 2.53: A reactive lymphocyte from a Gyr hybrid. The size of the cell is also increased.

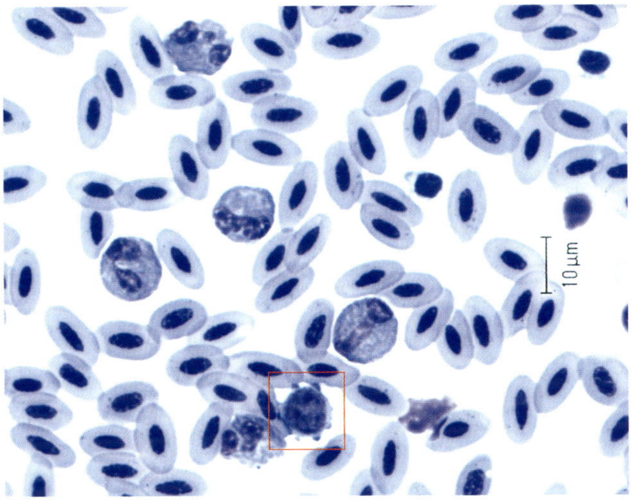

Figure 2.54: A lymphocyte with scalloped cytoplasmic borders and five normal heterophils of a Saker falcon.

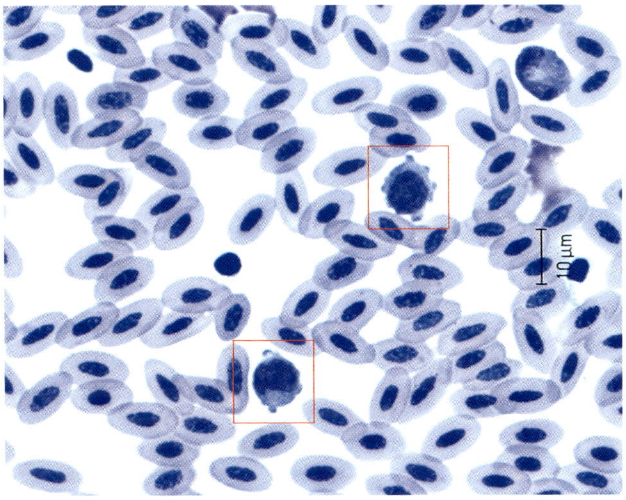

Figure 2.55: Two lymphocytes with scalloped cytoplasmic borders of a Saker falcon, one heterophil and two thrombocytes.

2

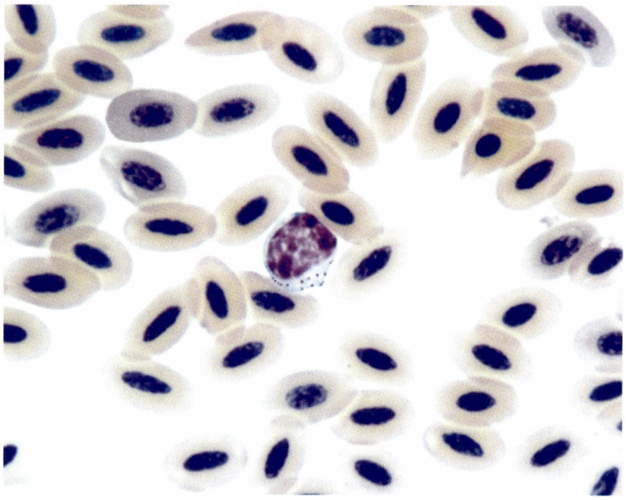

Figure 2.56: A lymphocyte with azurophilic granules of a Saker falcon (*Falco cherrug*).

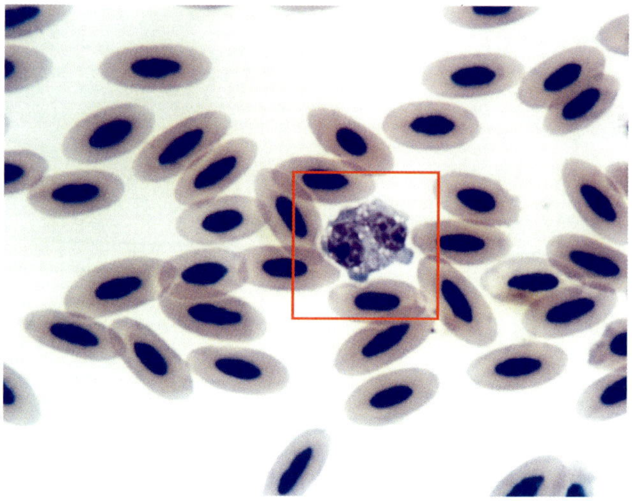

Figure 2.57: An eosinophil of a Saker falcon (*Falco cherrug*), note the granules are not stained properly, which gives an impression of numerous vacuoles within the cytoplasm.

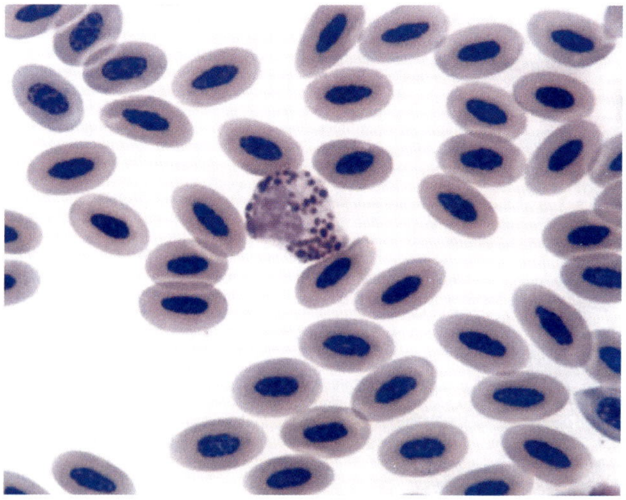

Figure 2.58: Although the central leukocyte possesses round granules like an eosinophil, it is in fact a heterophil with toxic granulation. This blood film is from a Gyr x Peregrine hybrid.

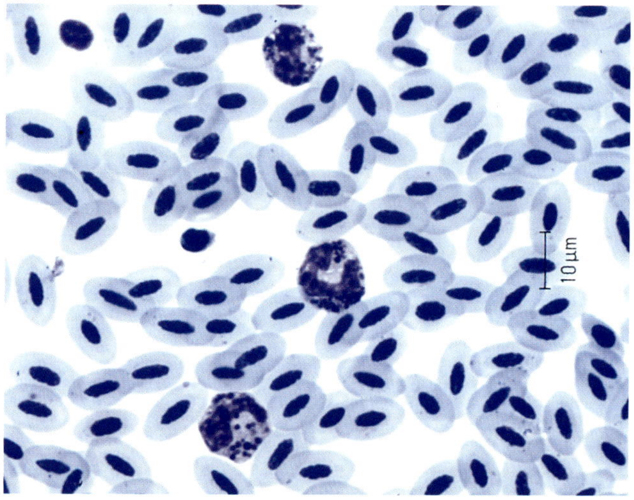

Figure 2.59: Three heterophils with toxic changes (+3) of a Gyr falcon.

Blood biochemistry

Biochemical parameters were conducted in a Hitachi 911 automatic analyser (Figure 2.60) using falcon plasma samples.

For this purpose, EDTA falcon blood samples were centrifuged following haematological analyses. Biochemical analyses were then performed on the plasma. Due to the small volume of blood received, a complete biochemical profile could not be obtained from every sample.

Blood biochemistry is essential to evaluate the birds' organ function, dehydration status, body condition, performance and inflammatory profile. Blood biochemical analysis is an important supplement to history and clinical examination in determining the health status of animals. Normal enzyme ranges in avian patients tend to run higher than in mammals and represent the normal turnover of tissue. Avian enzyme activities have been studied in selected species. However, very little is known about the function of each parameter in falcons. Overinterpretation of minor deviations from reference ranges should be avoided. This is particularly true for muscle and liver-derived enzymes. Table 2.13 shows the blood chemistry parameters measured in falcons. Important conclusions of avian tissue enzyme studies include the following:

AST (GOT)	present in all muscle types and liver tissue
CK	plentiful in skeleton muscle and also present in cardiac and smooth muscles, absent in liver
ALT (GPT)	present in a number of tissues
LDH	present in a number of tissues
GGT	activity is low in the avian liver

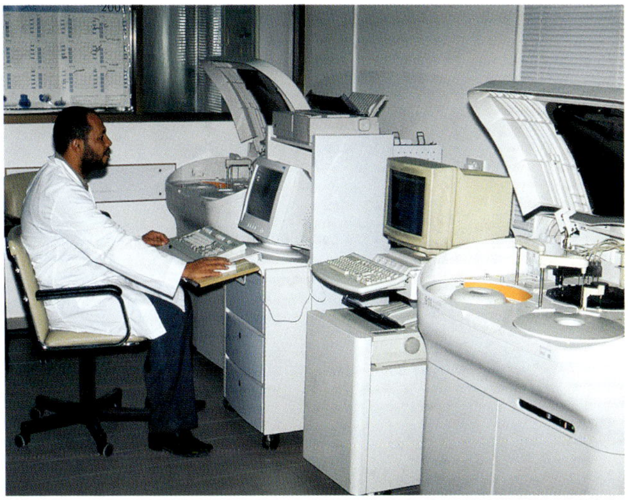

Figure 2.60: Blood biochemistry automated analyser.

2

Table 2.13: Blood chemistry parameters measured in falcons with explanation of their abbreviations and their SI Units

Abbreviations	Parameters	Conventional Units	Multiplication factors	SI Units
CK	Creatine kinase	IU/L	none	U/L
LDH	Lactate dehydrogenase	IU/L	none	U/L
ALT (GPT)	Alanine aminotransferase	IU/L	none	U/L
AST (GOT)	Aspartate aminotransferase	IU/L	none	U/L
GGT	γ-glutamyl transferase	IU/L	none	U/L
BUN	Blood urea nitrogen	mg/dl	x0.714	mmol/l
UA	Uric acid	mg/dl	x59.48	µmol/l
BA	Bile acids	–	–	µmol/l
TP	Total protein	g/dl	x10.0	g/l
ALB	Albumin	g/dl	x10.0	g/l
GLOB	Globulin	g/dl	x10.0	g/l
IRON	Iron	µg/dl	x0.179	µmol/l
CA	Calcium	mg/dl	x0.25	mmol/l
PHOS	Phosphorus	mg/dl	x0.323	mmol/l

2

Table 2.14: Clinical biochemistry assessment

Parameters	Abbreviations	Assessment
Creatine kinase	CK	A muscle specific enzyme which is elevated with muscle damage (striated and smooth muscle), excessive exercise, intramuscular injections, stress and nutritional myopathies in connection with Selenium/ Vit. E deficiencies. Plentiful in muscle and absent in liver. Marked elevations are specific for muscle damage. It has a short serum/plasma half-life. Levels peak after 6 to 12 hours and return to baseline 3 to 4 days later. Therefore, paired samples should be taken. Raised CK levels may result in a corresponding rise of AST, LDH and ALT values. CK is elevated in haemolysed samples.
Lactate dehydrogenase	LDH	Is not specific or sensitive for liver damage. Elevated values indicate either hepatocellular disease or muscle damage. LDH in avians possesses a shorter half-life than CK, and has no diagnostic advantage to AST. A disadvantage is the wide reference range (see Standard Deviation values). Haemolysis can markedly elevate LDH. LDH isoenzymes may be helpful in determining the source of elevated LDH activity.
Alanine aminotransferase	ALT (GPT)	Present in a number of tissues and therefore, not very organ specific. Elevated with skeletal and myocardial diseases as well as hepatopathy like hepatitis, hepatic necrosis and toxic liver damage. ALT is elevated in haemolysed samples.
Aspartate aminotransferase	AST (GOT)	Present in all muscle types, brain, kidney and liver tissues. Elevated with skeletal muscle damage as well as acute hepatopathy like viral hepatitis. Raised values are suspicious of liver disease, when CK is normal. Levels peak after 24 to 48 hours after a myopathic episode and only return to baseline after 10 to 14 days. Serial AST should be conducted to provide a useful guide to recovery from myopathy. AST is elevated in haemolysed samples.
γ-glutamyl transferase	GGT	Shows high specifity to avian liver tissue, but its sensitivity is low. This enzyme is controversially discussed in falcons. We found an increase when liver damage or clostridial enterotoxaemia occurred. It is increased when other liver-specific enzymes are also elevated.
Blood urea nitrogen	BUN	Urea is formed in the liver as a product of protein catabolism. Increase may be caused by pre-renal insufficiency due to haemorrhage, vomiting, diarrhoea, reduced water intake or due to post renal insufficiency after excessive protein intake.
Uric acid	UA	UA is the major end product of nitrogen metabolism, and is only elevated if more than 70 % of renal function is impaired. Hyperuricaemia occurs with high protein diet, starvation, severe tissue necrosis, lead intoxication, urinary obstruction, nephritis, nephrocalcinosis and A hypovitaminosis. If UA cannot be dissolved in plasma or serum, gout may develop.
Bile acids	BA	Very specific and sensitive for the diagnosis of hepatic diseases. BA offers an indication of hepatic function. This parameter is therefore of greater value than ALT and AST. BA are produced in the liver, excreted in the bile, reabsorbed by the intestines into the portal circulation, and removed from the blood by hepatocytes (entero-hepatic circulation). A 24 h fast is recommended for BA testing because of the digestive physiology of birds. Increases of BA are suggestive of: abnormal hepatic uptake, bile acid storage, excretion or hepatic perfusion. BA cannot be measured using the automated chemistry analyser, but in a spectro-photometer with a filter of 530 mm (e.g. Ultrospec 3000, Pharmacia Biotech, Uppsala, Sweden).

Table 2.14: Clinical biochemistry assessment (continued)

Parameters	Abbreviations	Assessment
Total protein	TP	Elevations are associated with dehydration, acute and chronic inflammation. Decreases are associated with blood loss, emaciation, maldigestion, enteropathy, hepatopathy and anaemias.
Albumin	ALB	An elevation is seen with haemoconcentration and dehydration, a decrease is observed with protein-loosing enteropathy, e.g. salmonellosis, parasitosis, chronic malabsorption. A decrease is also seen with liver diseases, because the liver is the sole site of albumin synthesis.
Globulin	GLOB	Elevations are associated with infectious diseases, dehydration and inflammation; decreases are associated with protein losing enteropathy (in conjunction with hypoalbuminaemia), failure of passive immunity transfer and genetic disorders.
Iron	IRON	Iron is decreased with mineral imbalances and malabsorption syndrome. Microcytic, hypochromic anaemia and reticulocytosis may develop.
Calcium	CA	Control of CA metabolism is mediated by parathormone (PTH), calcitonin and vitamin D_3. CA is important for bone metabolism, neural and muscle cells and for the development of egg shell. Approximately, one-third to one-half of plasma CA is bound to albumin. Therefore, the plasma Ca concentration is affected by the plasma albumin concentration. Hypocalcaemia may induce cramps, seizure and convulsions, and it occurs with: hypoalbuminaemia, dietary CA and vitamin D_3 deficiency, excessive dietary phosphorus. Hypercalcaemia may be associated with bone tumors, Vit. D_3-hypervitaminosis and hyperparathyroidism
Phosphorus	PHOS	PHOS is primarily regulated via renal excretion stimulated by PTH. Hyperphosphotaemia: severe renal disease (reduced glomerular filtration), hypervitaminosis D_3, excessive dieatary phosphorus. Hypophosphotaemia: hypovitaminosis D_3, malabsorption, starvation, long-term corticosteroid therapy and malabsorption syndrome.

Table 2.15: Significance of enzyme elevations

CK	Recent muscle damage, sample haemolysis
LDH	Recent liver or muscle damage, sample haemolysis
ALT (GPT)	Infrequent with hepatocellular damage, sample haemolysis
AST (GOT)	Liver or muscle damage, sample haemolysis
GGT	Liver damage, sample haemolysis

Table 2.16: Clinical interpretation of falcon enzyme profile combinations

Normal CK, LDH, AST	No liver or muscle damage
Elevated CK, LDH, AST	Skeletal or cardiac muscle damage
Normal CK; Elevated LDH and AST	Most probably hepatocellular damage
Normal AST; Elevated LDH and CK	Skeletal or Cardiac muscle damage
Normal LDH and CK; Elevated AST	Most probably hepatic damage
Normal CK and AST; Elevated LDH	Sample haemolysis or processing error

2

Table 2.17: Plasma chemistry values of clinically normal falcons

Parameters	N	Mean ± SD	Conventional Units	Mean ± SD	SI Units
CK	519	640 ± 210	U/L	640 ± 210	U/L
LDH	253	1028 ± 385	U/L	1028 ± 385	U/L
ALT	353	64.8 ± 28.9	U/L	64.8 ± 28.9	U/L
AST	353	93.1 ± 44.6	U/L	93.1 ± 44.6	U/L
GGT	247	14.0 ± 6.3	U/L	14.0 ± 6.3	U/L
BUN	159	6.6 ± 2.5	mg/dl	4.7 ± 1.8	mmol/l
UA	328	8.2 ± 4.5	mg/dl	487 ± 267	µmol/l
BA	631	22.3 ± 4.7	µmol/l	22.3 ± 4.7	µmol/l
TP	405	2.84 ± 0.65	g/dl	28.4 ± 6.5	g/l
ALB	405	1.04 ± 0.19	g/dl	10.4 ± 1.9	g/l
GLOB	405	1.80 ± 0.46	g/dl	18.0 ± 4.6	g/l
IRON	333	33.8 ± 20.8	mg/dl	6.1 ± 3.7	µmol/l
CA	134	9.7 ± 1.3	mg/dl	2.4 ± 0.3	mmol/l
PHOS	181	2.3 ± 0.9	mg/dl	0.7 ± 0.3	mmol/l

Table 2.18: Plasma chemistry reference values of selected species of raptors from the literature

Assay	Lanner falcon[1]	Gyr falcon[2]	Peregrine falcon[1,2]	Saker falcon[1,3]	Merlin[1]	Gyr Falcon[4]
	Falco biarmicus	*Falco rusticolus*	*Falco peregrinus*	*Falco cherrug*	*Falco columbarius*	*Falco rusticolus*
	N=26	N=12	N=55, 14	N=38	N=39	N=53
Total protein (g/l)*	33–42	28.9	25–40	27–36	27.5–39	25.0 (8.7)
Albumin (g/l)	9.6–16	7.3	8.3–12.5	9–12.3	8.6–16.1	11.8 (1.7)
Globulin (g/l)	21.2–28.8	–	16–28	18–28	17.2–25	–
A:G ratio	0.44–0.57	–	0.4–0.55	0.45–0.57	0.47–0.58	–
Urea (mmol/l)	1.3–2.7	–	0.9–2.8	0.5–2.6	–	3.6 (2.2)
Creatinine (μmol/l)	37–75	–	41–91	23–75	16–50	38 (14)
Uric acid (μmol/l)	318–709	828.56	326–675	320–785	174–800	370 (170)
Bile acids (μmol/l)	–	–	20–118	20–90	–	–
ALT (SGPT) (u/l)	–	–	15–51	36–55	–	135 (125)
ALP (u/l)	180–510	257	97–350	285–450	54–310	–
GGT (u/l)	–	–	0–7	0.8–5.9	–	–
AST (SGOT) (u/l)	30–118	97	50–105	45–95	50–125	149 (110)
CK (u/l)	350–650	402	357–850	355–651	521–807	–
LDH (u/l)	434–897	–	625–1210	551–765	320–630	1917 (879)
Glucose (mmol/l)	11–15	17.65	11–16	12–14	9–12	20.4 (1.7)
Cholesterol (mmol/l)	3–8.8	–	3.9–10.5	4.5–8.6	3–7.8	5.44 (1.03)
Inorg phosphate (mmol/l)	0.68–2	–	0.77–2.1	0.72–2.16	0.95–1.79	–
Calcium (mmol/l)	2.07–2.45	2.40	2.1–2.56	2.15–2.61	2–2.45	2.30 (0.27)
Sodium (mmol/l)	152–164	160	153–164	154–161	155–170	154 (12)
Potassium (mmol/l)	1–2.1	1.99	0.9–1.7	0.8–2.3	1–1.8	3.1 (0.9)
Chloride (mmol/l)	–	125	117–127	114–125	–	124 (8)

▶▶

2

Table 2.18: Plasma chemistry reference values of selected species of raptors from the literature (continued)

Assay	Lanner falcon[1]	Gyr falcon[2]	Peregrine falcon[1,2]	Saker falcon[1,3]	Merlin[1]	Gyr Falcon[4]
	Falco biarmicus	*Falco rusticolus*	*Falco peregrinus*	*Falco cherrug*	*Falco columbarius*	*Falco rusticolus*
	N=26	N=12	N=55, 14	N=38	N=39	N=53
Amylase (u/l)	–	–	–	–	–	86 (116)
Bilirubin (µmol/l)	–	–	78.15	8.55–27.53	–	4.6 (1.7)
Blood urea nitrogen (mmol/l)	–	3.33	2.32	–	–	–
Phosphorus (mg/dl)	–	3.57	3.35	–	–	1.52 (0.40 mmol/l)
Triglycerides (mmol/l)	–	–	–	0.79–1.25	–	1.02 (0.27)

* Conversion Table for SI units see Table 2.13

1 JENNINGS IV: Appendix 8.1 Haematology and clinical chemistry values. In Beynon PH, Forbes NA, Harcourt-Brown NH (ed): Manual of raptors, pigeons and waterfowl. British Small Animal Veterinary Association, Cheltenham, UK, 1996, 75–78

2 ALTMAN RB, CLUBB SL, DORRESTEIN GM, QUESENBERRY K (eds): Appendix I, Avian Medicine and Surgery. Philadelphia: WB Saunders, 1997

3 SAMOUR JH, D'ALOIA M-A: Normal blood chemistry of saker falcon (Falco cherrug). Avian Pathology 25, 175–178, 1996

4 LIERZ M: Plasma chemistry reference values for gyrfalcons (Falco rusticolus). The Vet. Rec. 153, 182–183, 2003

Chapter 3

Viral Diseases

Paramyxovirus-1 infection

Falcon Herpesvirus infection

Falconpox

Influenza

Paramyxovirus-1 infection, pox, herpesvirus and influenza are the most important viral diseases in falcons. For the facilitation of the reader, the column of the reference values has also been included into all following tables of diseased falcons. In these tables significant changes in haematology and biochemistry values are indicated by arrows. Haematological results show a decrease in nearly all values, except for lymphocytes which are elevated, and an increase in enzymes and minerals. However, even in herpesvirus infection, which is the most devastating falcon viral infection, WBC does not drop very low, but falcons with values below 5.0×10^9/l have a grave prognosis. A very significant rise is observed in AST, ALT and BA. A separate haematology and biochemistry Table (Table 3.3) has been produced for 7 herpesvirus infected falcons, because many values are even more altered in comparison to the other viral infections. Due to the severe destruction of the liver parenchyma, blood values for BA from the herpesvirus infected falcons regularly exceed 200 µmol/l. Total protein (TP) is also elevated in viral infections most probably due to tissue damage, and the increase in globulin concentration.

Haematological pictures of falcons with viral infections

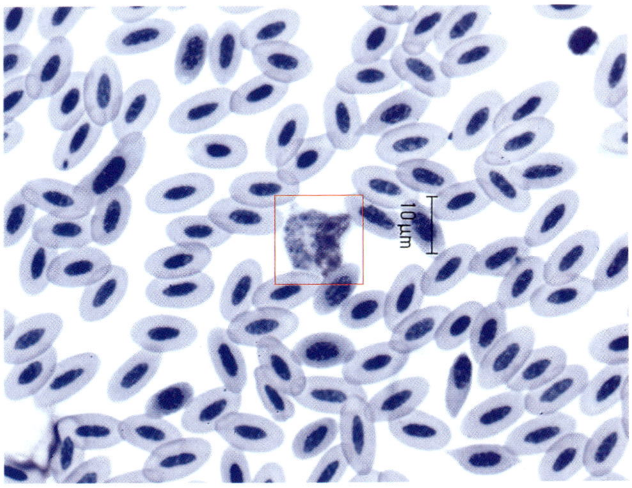

Figure 3.1: One toxic heterophil (+2). Dark blue spots (central body) are visible in the toxic granula. This Gyr falcon had a herpesvirus infection.

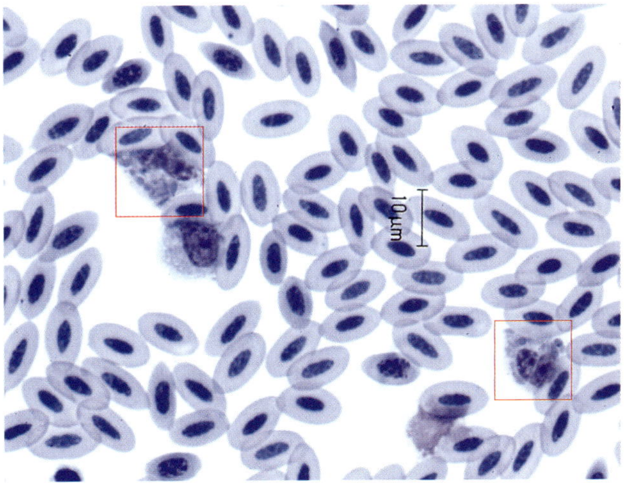

Figure 3.2: Two toxic heterophils (+1) and one monocyte. This Gyr falcon suffered from inclusion body hepatitis caused by herpesvirus infection.

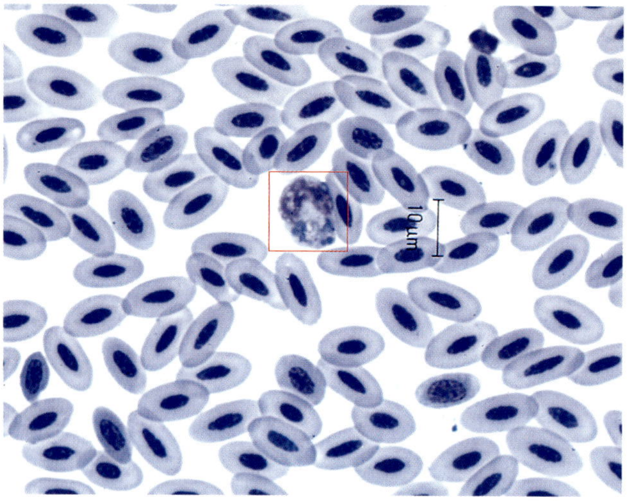

Figure 3.3: A toxic heterophil (+3) from a Gyr falcon with herpesvirus infection (RBC 2.48 x 10^{12}/l, WBC 4.8 x 10^{9}/l, 32 % heterophils, 58 % lymphocytes, 10 % monocytes).

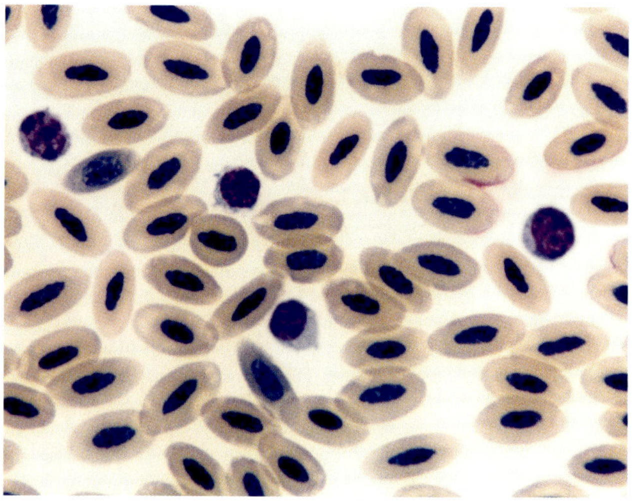

Figure 3.4: Lymphocytosis in a Saker falcon (*Falco cherrug*), with Paramyxovirus-1 infection. Lymphocytosis develops with a viral infection. In this picture four lymphocytes are visible. This Saker falcon showed a WBC 6.34 x 10^{9}/l with 64 % lymphocytes, 30 % heterophils and 6 % monocytes.

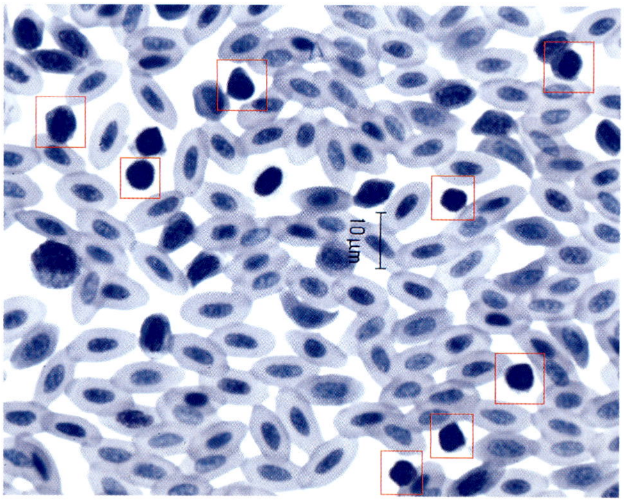

Figure 3.5: A Saker falcon with PMV-1, which had developed CNS signs. This picture shows eight small lymphocytes (lymphocytosis), a monocyte and two thrombocytes.

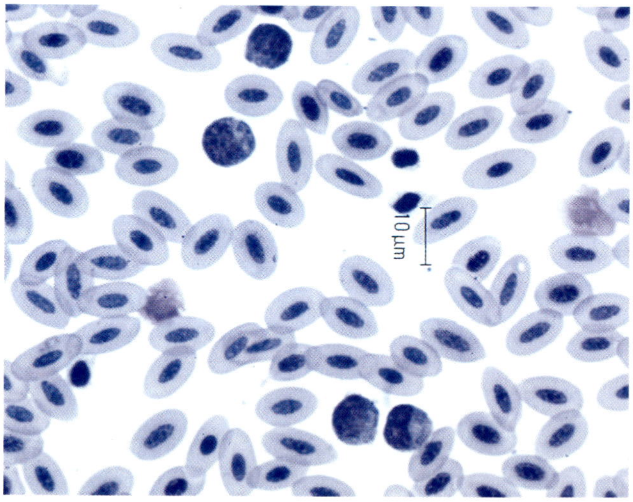

Figure 3.6: Four normal monocytes and three normal thrombocytes. This Peregrine falcon suffered from Influenzavirus infection (monocytosis). Monocyte levels above 7 % suggest chronic infection and require a complete check-up.

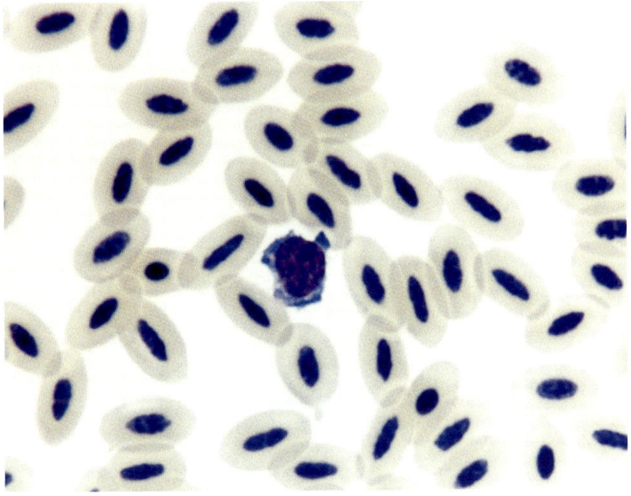

Figure 3.7: A large reactive lymphocyte: The nucleus is round, centrally located and dark purple in colour. The cytoplasm is deeply basophilic. This Gyr falcon (*Falco rusticolus*) suffered from viral inclusion body hepatitis.

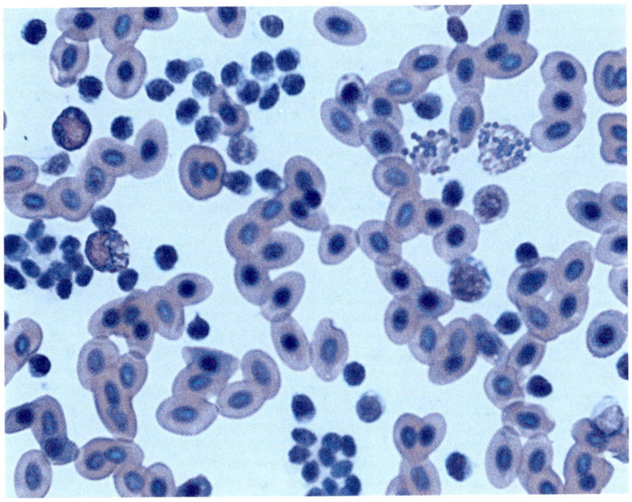

Figure 3.8: Lymphocytosis in a Gyr falcon with falconpox infection. In chronic pox cases, the lymphocyte count may exceed 60 %.

Table 3.1: Haematology and biochemistry values of falcons suffering from viral diseases

Para-meters	SI Units	N	Mean ± SD Diseased Falcons	Mean ± SD Reference Values
RBC	$x10^{12}/l$	35	▼ **2.84** ± 0.42	3.21 ± 0.30
HB	g/dl	35	▼ **13.33** ± 2.13	14.95 ± 1.39
HCT	l/l	35	▼ **0.40** ± 0.7	0.45 ± 0.04
MCV	fl	35	140.84 ± 7.36	139.85 ± 6.33
MCH	pg	35	46.94 ± 2.67	46.42 ± 2.55
WBC	$x10^{9}/l$	35	▼ **7.04** ± 3.64	9.64 ± 3.96
HETERO	%	35	▼ **47.20** ± 14.19	59.80 ± 12.87
LYMPHO	%	35	▲ **48.07** ± 11.68	34.84 ± 12.88
MONO	%	35	4.43 ± 2.74	4.46 ± 2.77
EOS	%	35	0.00	0.43
BASO	%	35	0.00	0.16
CK	U/L	31	▲ **758** ± 207	640 ± 210
LDH	U/L	31	969 ± 281	1028 ± 385
ALT	U/L	31	▲ **97.7** ± 22.8	64.8 ± 28.9
AST	U/L	31	▲ **193.5** ± 80.1	93.1 ± 44.6
GGT	U/L	31	11.4 ± 5.2	14.0 ± 6.3
BUN	mmol/l	20	▲ **9.5** ± 2.1	4.7 ± 1.8
UA	µmol/l	20	▲ **656** ± 280	487 ± 267
BA	µmol/l	25	▲ **176.5** ± 71.4	22.3 ± 4.7
TP	g/l	20	▲ **37.8** ± 7.1	28.4 ± 6.5
ALB	g/l	20	10.0 ± 1.6	10.4 ± 1.9
GLOB	g/l	20	▲ **27.8** ± 7.3	18.0 ± 4.6
IRON	µmol/l	20	▲ **14.7** ± 4.8	6.1 ± 3.7
CA	mmol/l	20	2.3 ± 0.6	2.4 ± 0.3
PHOS	mmol/l	20	▲ **1.2** ± 0.1	0.7 ± 0.3

3

3

Paramyxovirus-1 infection

Table 3.2: The nine classified serotypes of avian paramyxoviruses

PMV-1	Newcastle disease virus
PMV-2	Chicken/California/Yucaipa/56
PMV-3	Turkey/Wisconsin/68
PMV-4	Duck/Hong Kong/D3/75
PMV-5	Budgerigar/Japan/Kunitachi/75
PMV-6	Duck/Hong Kong/199/77
PMV-7	Dove/Tennessee/4/75
PMV-8	Goose/Delaware/1053/76
PMV-9	Duck/New York/22/78

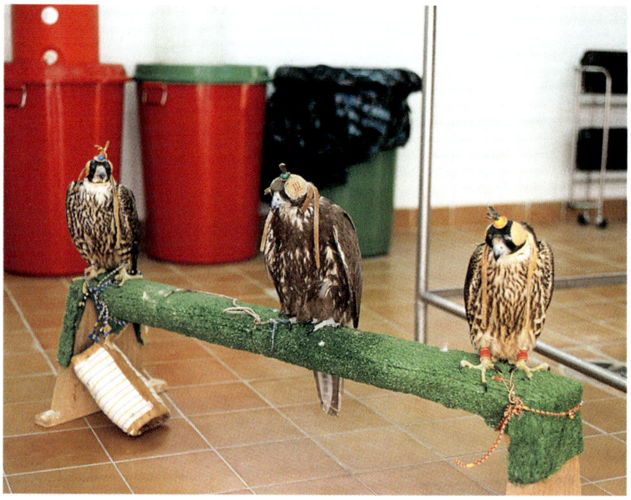

Figure 3.9: Three Saker falcons *(Falco cherrug)* suffering from PMV-1 infection. The predominant signs are nervous system abnormalities with ataxia, head tics, tremors, wing and leg paralysis, and torticollis. So far only PMV-1 has been isolated from falcons.

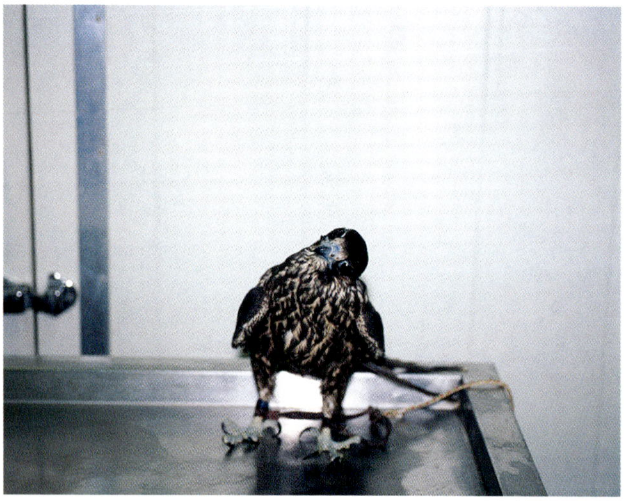

Figure 3.10: Saker falcon with torticollis.

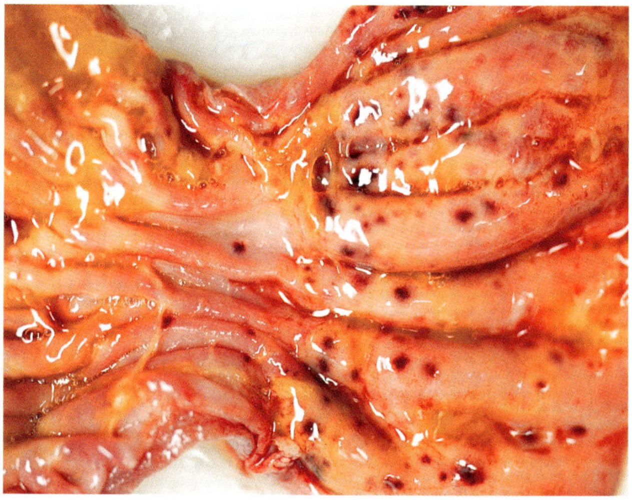

Figure 3.11: Petechial haemorrhages in the proventriculus of a Gyr falcon. This is pathognomonic for the gastro-intestinal form of PMV-1 infection.

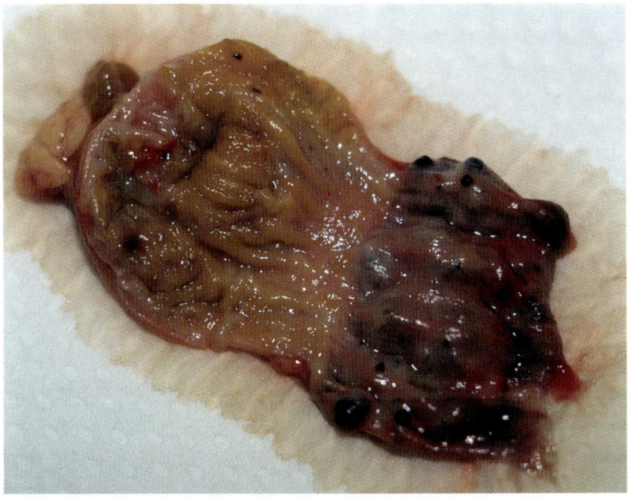

Figure 3.12: Gizzard of a Saker falcon. Petechial haemorrhages in the submucosa caused by PMV-1.

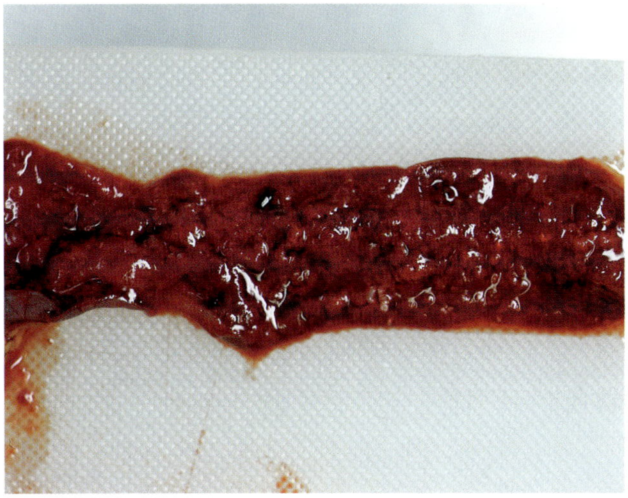

Figure 3.13: The enteric form of PMV-1 infection: Haemorrhagic enteritis causing bloody diarrhoea in a Gyr falcon. This form of PMV-1 infection is rare in falcons and may be confused with salmonellosis or clostridial enterotoxaemia.

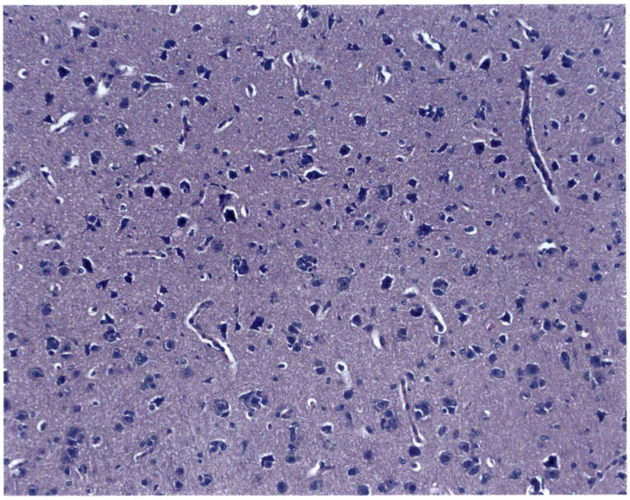

Figure 3.14: Encephalitis of the brain stem of a Peregrine falcon: Marked focal gliosis with neuronal degeneration (shrunken, basophilic cells). No inclusion bodies are visible. This lesion is not pathognomonic for PMV-1, but often observed in falcon PMV-1. HE stain.

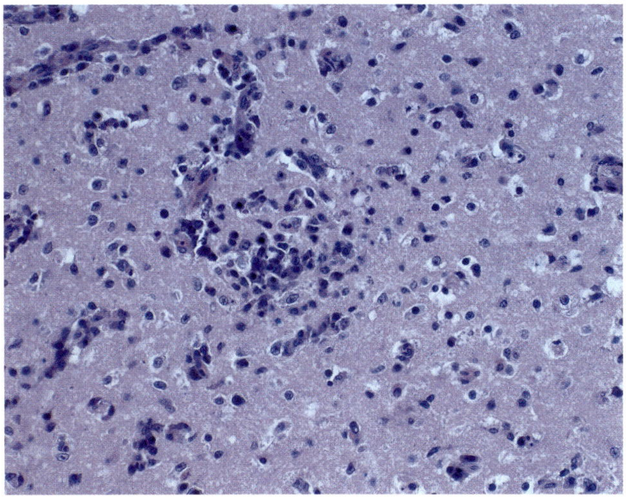

Figure 3.15: Encephalitis of the brain stem of a Gyr hybrid: Focal non-suppurative inflammation with early stage demyelinisation. In most cases only mild encephalitis is observed. HE stain.

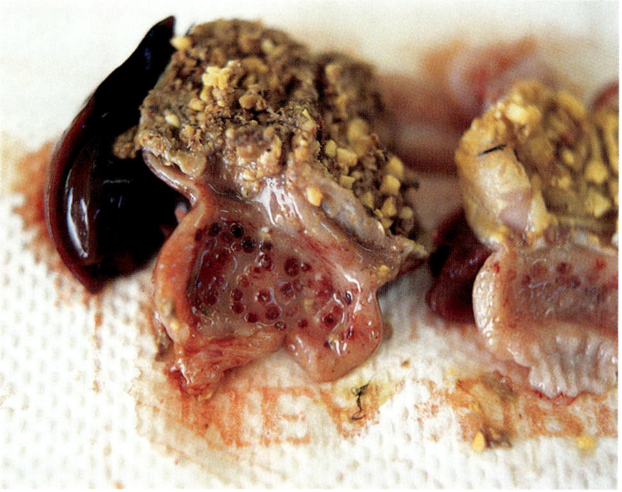

Figure 3.16: Chicken with Newcastle Disease (ND): Petechial haemorrhages within the gizzard. Falcons contract their PMV-1 infections through ingesting infected avians like chickens, quails and pigeons.

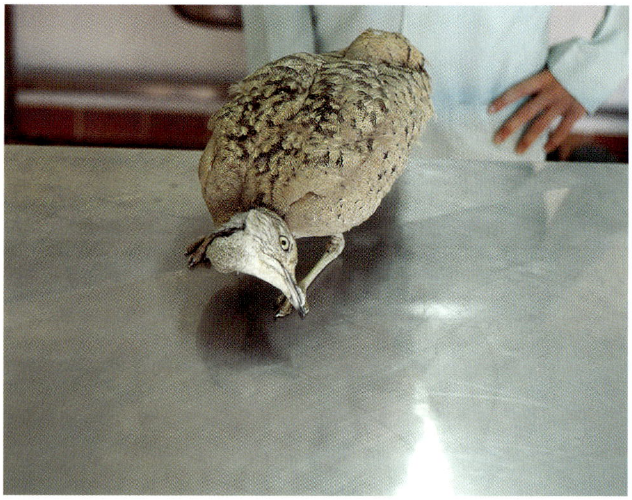

Figure 3.17: Houbara Bustard (*Chlamydotis undulata macqueenii)* with PMV-1 infection showing torticollis.

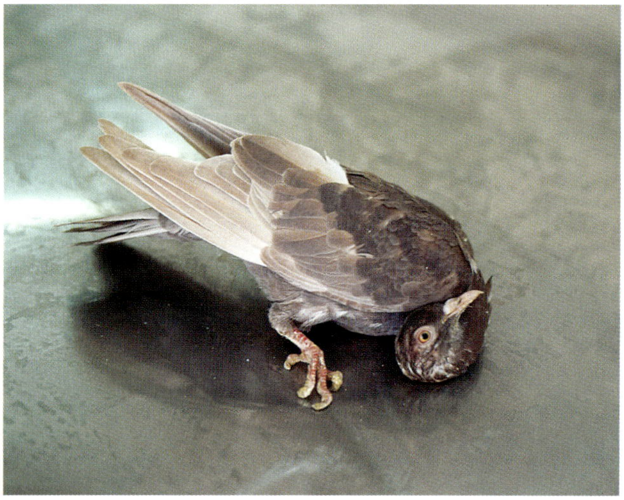

Figure 3.18: ND in a domestic pigeon *(Columba livia)* showing torticollis.

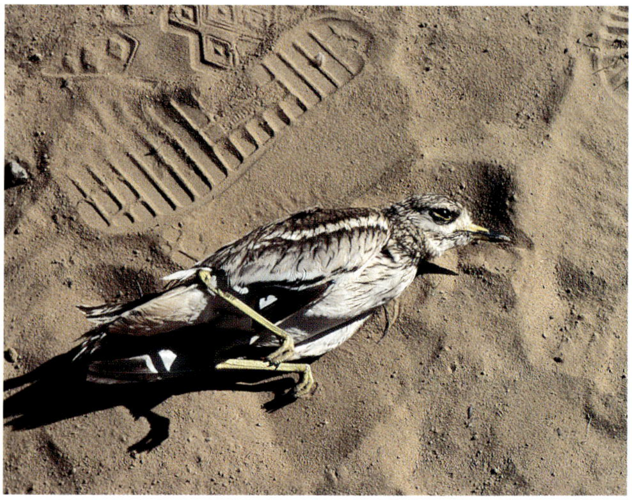

Figure 3.19: ND in a Stone Curlew *(Burhinus oedicnemus).*

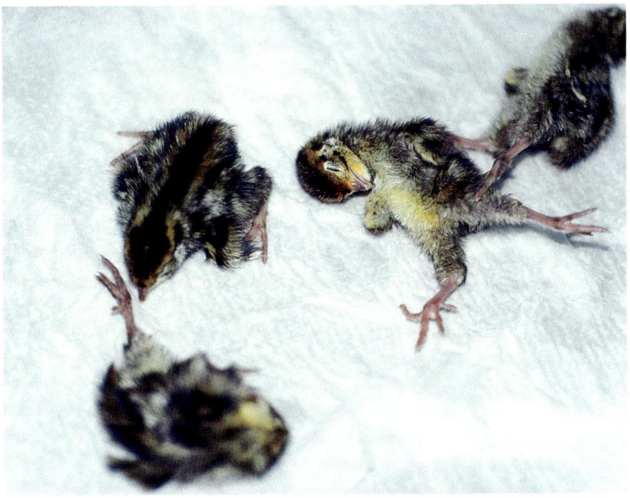

Figure 3.20: ND in one-day-old quails *(Coturnix coturnix)*.

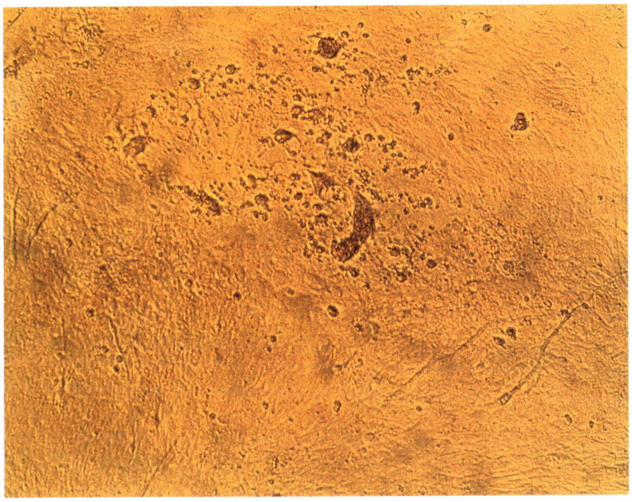

Figure 3.21: Cytopathogenic effect (CPE) of the PMV-1 virus on chicken embryo fibroblasts (CEF), 3 days after inoculation.

Falcon Herpesvirus infection

Table 3.3: Haematology and biochemistry values of seven falcons suffering from herpesvirus infection

Para-meters	SI Units	Mean ± SD Diseased Falcons	Mean ± SD Reference Values
RBC	$x10^{12}/l$	▼ **2.46** ± 0.56	3.21 ± 0.30
HB	g/dl	▼ **12.33** ± 3.10	14.95 ± 1.39
HCT	l/l	▼ **0.37** ± 0.07	0.45 ± 0.04
MCV	fl	▲ **150.41** ± 6.36	139.85 ± 6.33
MCH	pg	▲ **50.12** ± 2.78	46.42± 2.55
WBC	$x10^{9}/l$	▼ **6.34** ± 2.21	9.64 ± 3.96
HETERO	%	▼ **45.20** ± 15.31	59.80 ± 12.87
LYMPHO	%	▲ **51.32** ± 10.41	34.84 ± 12.88
MONO	%	3.42 ± 2.01	4.46 ± 2.77
EOS	%	0.00	0.43
BASO	%	0.00	0.16
CK	U/L	▲ **896** ± 311	640 ± 210
LDH	U/L	1110 ± 410	1028 ± 385
ALT	U/L	▲ **212.8** ± 33.2	64.8 ± 28.9
AST	U/L	▲ **495.7** ± 160.3	93.1 ± 44.6
GGT	U/L	▲ **116.2** ± 16.8	14.0 ± 6.3
BUN	mmol/l	▲ **13.4** ± 2.8	4.7 ± 1.8
UA	µmol/l	▲ **631** ± 382	487 ± 267
BA	µmol/l	> 200	22.3 ± 4.7
TP	g/l	nd *	28.4 ± 6.5
ALB	g/l	nd	10.4 ± 1.9
GLOB	g/l	nd	18.0 ± 4.6
IRON	µmol/l	nd	6.1 ± 3.7
CA	mmol/l	2.5 ± 0.4	2.4 ± 0.3
PHOS	mmol/l	▲ **4.6** ± 2.1	0.7 ± 0.3

* nd = not done

3

3

Table 3.4: Classification of the avian herpesviruses

Serogroup	Disease	Virus		Subfamily
1	Marek's disease of chicken	Gallid	Ga HV-2	Gammaherpesvirinae
2	Duck plague – viral enteritis	Anatid	An HV-1	Alphaherpesvirinae
3	Infectious laryngotracheitis of chicken	Gallid	Ga HV-1	Alphaherpesvirinae
4	Pacheco's disease of psittacines	Psittacid	Ps HV-1	nc
5	Pacheco's disease of psittacines	Psittacid	Ps HV-2	nc
6	Pacheco's disease of psittacines	Psittacid	Ps HV-3	nc
7	Inclusion of body hepatitis of pigeons	Columbid	Co HV-1	nc
8	Inclusion of body hepatitis of pigeons	Columbid	Co HV-2	nc
9	None? HV of cormorants	Phalacrocoracid	Ph HV-1	nc
10	Inclusion body hepatitis of cranes	Gruid	Gr HV-1	nc
11	Inclusion body hepatitis of storks	Ciconiid	Ci HV-1	nc
–	Inclusion body hepatitis of falcons	Falconid	Fa HV-1	nc
–	Inclusion body hepatitis of eagles	Accipitrid	Ac HV-1	nc
–	Inclusion body hepatitis of owls	Strigid	St HV-1	nc
–	Inclusion body hepatitis of quails	Perdicid	Pe HV-1	nc
–	None? HV of turkeys	Meleagrid	Me HV-1	Gammaherpesvirinae
–	None? HV of penguins	Sphenicid	Sp HV-1	nc

nc = not classified

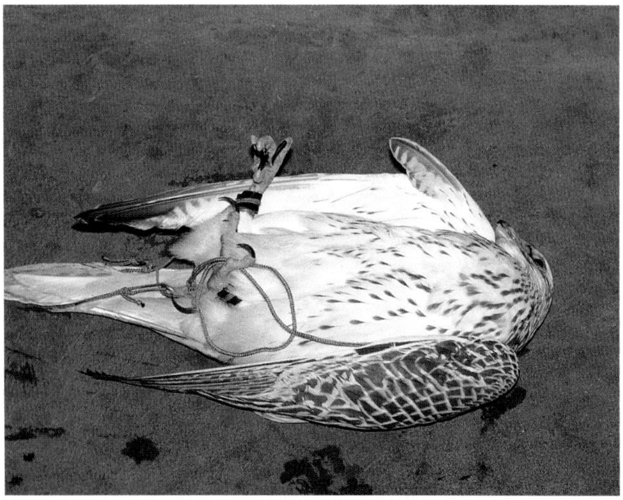

Figure 3.22: All falcon species are affected by ›inclusion body hepatitis‹, but Gyr falcons *(Falco rusticolus)* are extremely sensitive to the herpesvirus. The falconid herpesvirus (FHV-1), the owl herpesvirus (Strigid, StHV-1) and the pigeon herpesvirus (PHV-1) are serologically and genetically related.

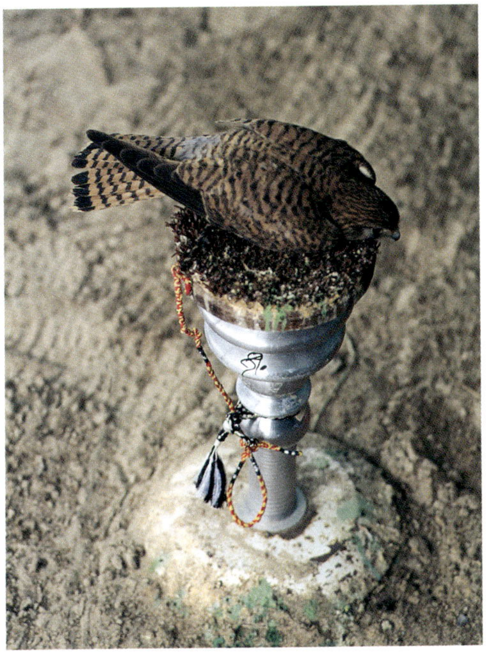

Figure 3.23: A Common Kestrel *(Falco tinnunculus)* with FHV-1 infection. The falcon is extremely weak and anorectic and excretes green mutes due to the destruction of the liver parenchyma by the virus. The source of infection is mainly pigeons which are fed to hunting falcons.

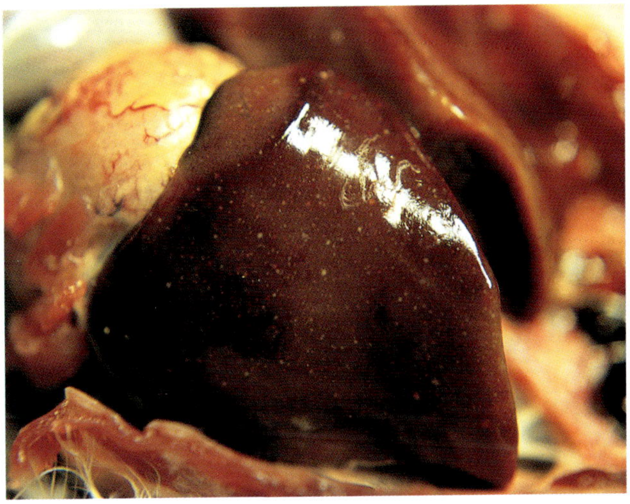

Figure 3.24: Multiple miliar necrosis of the liver in a Common Kestrel caused by FHV-1. The liver and the spleen are the target organs. The disease is fatal.

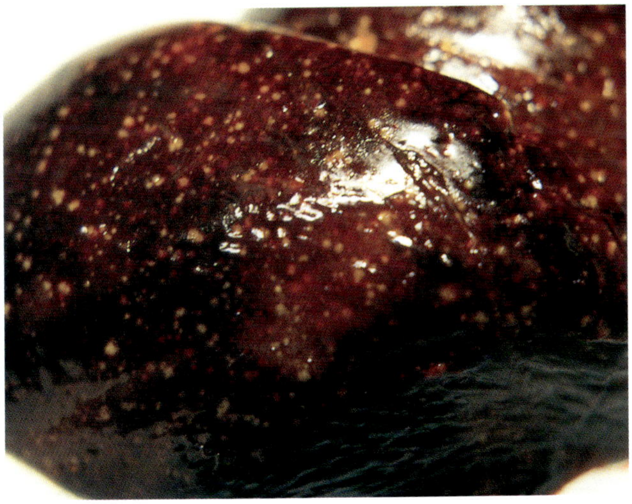

Figure 3.25: Severe inclusion body hepatitis in a Gyr falcon.

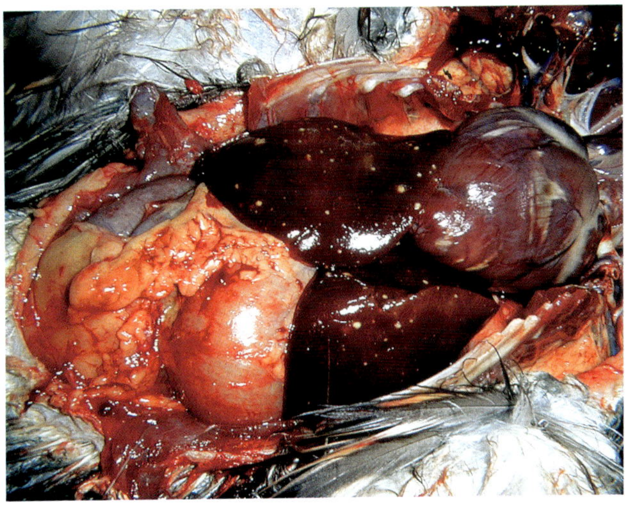

Figure 3.26: Herpesvirus infection in a Saker falcon caused degeneration of heart muscle.

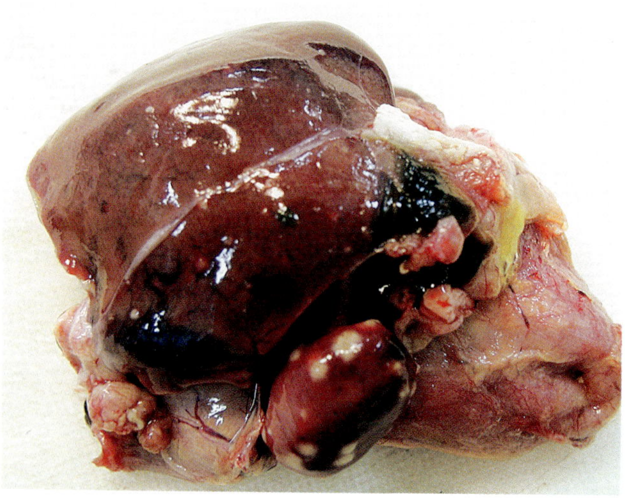

Figure 3.27: Miliar necrosis in spleen and liver.

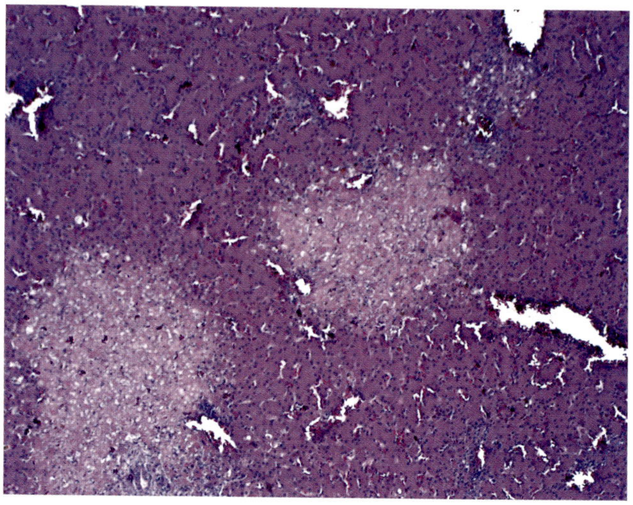

Figure 3.28: Miliar necrosis in the liver of a Gyr falcon. HE stain.

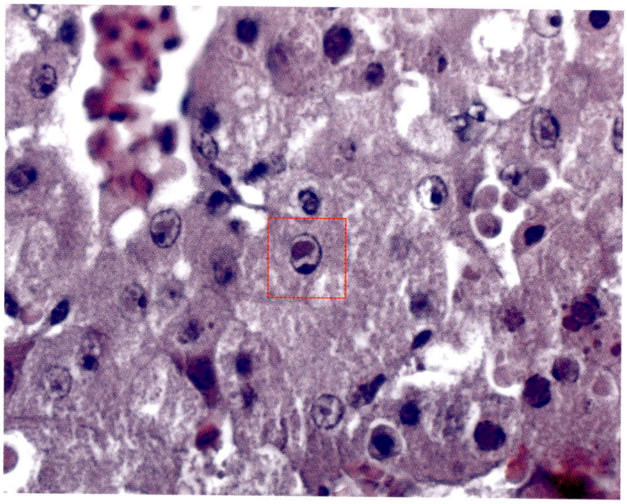

Figure 3.29: Herpesvirus inclusion body in a liver section of a *Falco rusticolus*. HE stain.

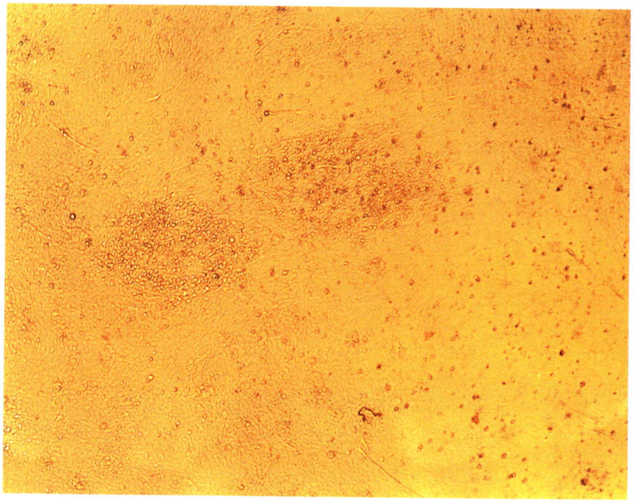

Figure 3.30: Cytopathic effect (CPE) on primary chicken embryo fibroblasts (CEF) three days after infection with FHV-1. An attenuated falcon herpes virus vaccine (DuFaHe) has been developed at Central Veterinary Research Laboratory (CVRL) to protect falcons from inclusion body hepatitis.

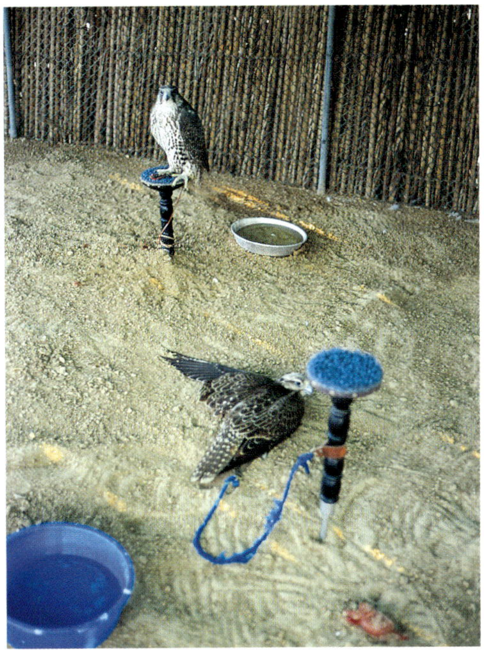

Figure 3.31: A moribund control (non-vaccinated and challenged) Gyr hybrid (foreground) and one vaccinated and challenged healthy falcon in the back during a (DuFaHe) vaccination trial. The efficacy and safety of DuFaHe has been evaluated in different vaccination trials.

Falconpox

Table 3.5: Classification of the Avipox viruses

Family	Poxviridae
Subfamily	Chordopoxvirinae
Genus	Avipox virus

Species		**Tentative species in the genus APV**	
Canarypox virus	CNPV	Crowpox virus	CRPV
Fowlpox virus	FWPV	Peacockpox virus	PKPV
Juncopox virus	JNPV	Penguinpox virus	PEPV
Mynahpox virus	MYPV	Falconpox virus	FAPV
Pigeonpox virus	PGPV	Houbarapox virus	HOPV
Psittacinepox virus	PSPV	Stone Curlewpox virus	SCPV
Quailpoxvirus	QUPV		
Sparrowpox virus	SRPV		
Starlingpox virus	SLPV		
Turkeypox virus	TKPV		

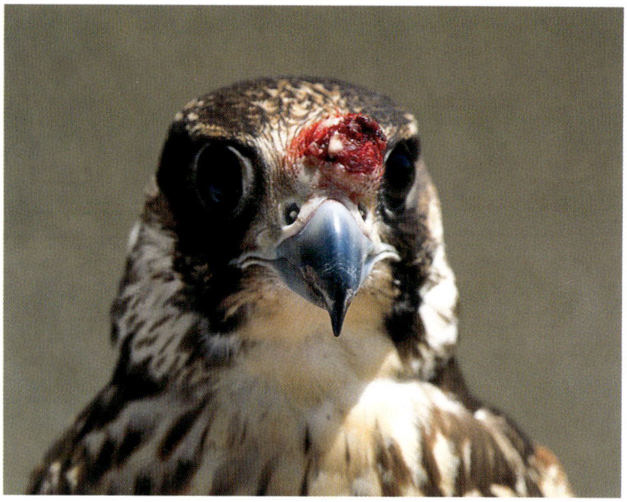

Figure 3.32: A typical pox lesion above the cere of a Peregrine falcon *(Falco peregrinus)*. The poxvirus is spread by biting insect vectors. Pox in falcons in the United Arab Emirates is of major clinical significance, because in the majority of cases, severe skin lesions are observed when falcons return from hunting expeditions to the Middle East countries.

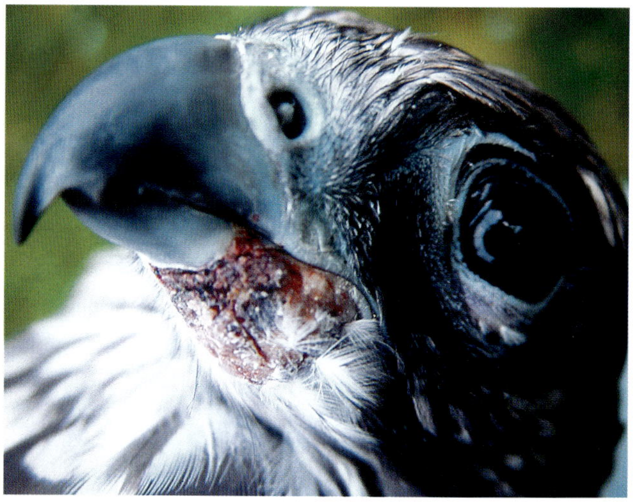

Figure 3.33 a: Pox lesions in a Saker falcon: Under the beak.

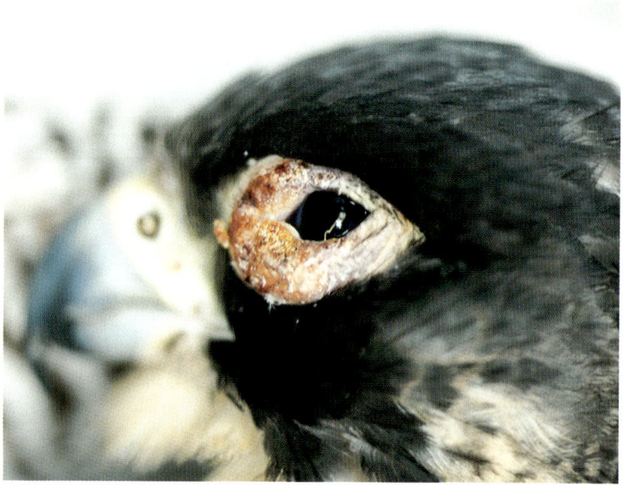

Figure 3.33 b: Pox lesions in a Saker falcon: On the eyelids.

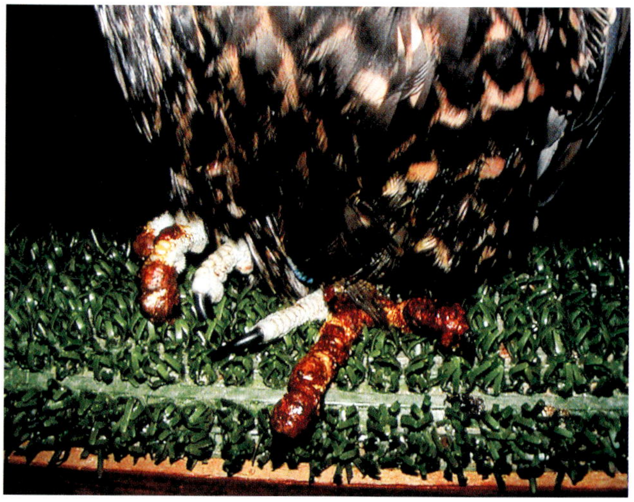

Figure 3.33 c: Pox lesions in a Saker falcon: On the feet.

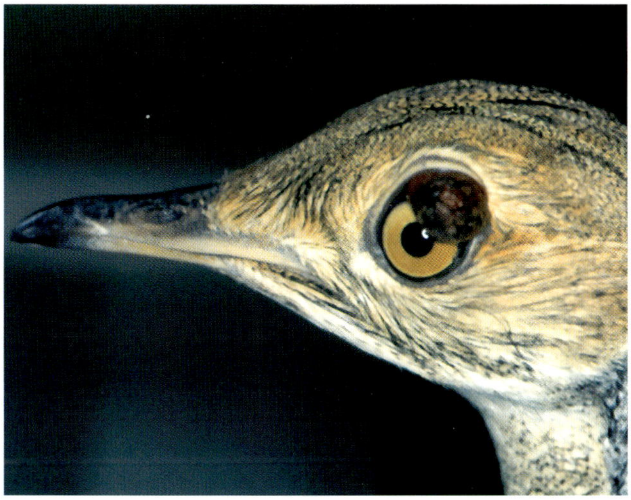

Figure 3.34: Pox lesions on the upper eyelid of a Houbara Bustard (*Chlamydotis undulata*).

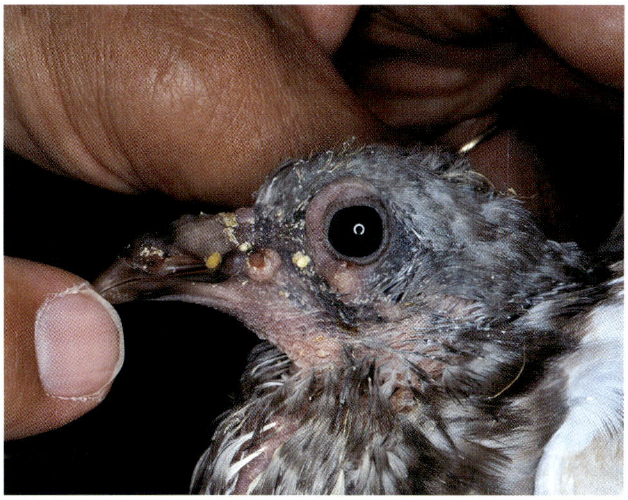

Figure 3.35: Pox lesions around the face of a domestic pigeon *(Columba livia).*

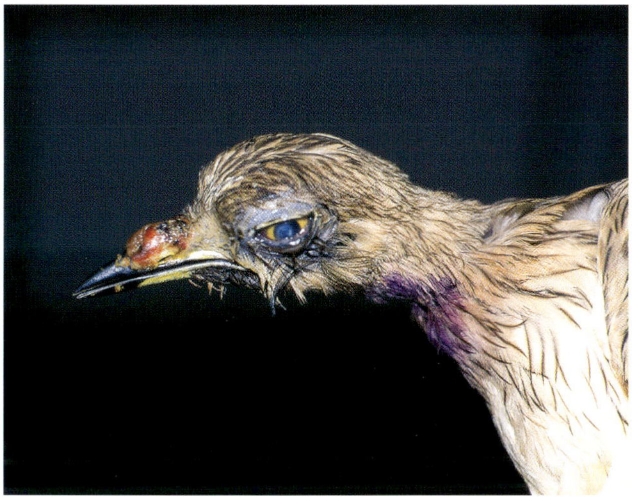

Figure 3.36: Pox lesions on the cere of a Stone Curlew *(Burhinus oedicnemus).*

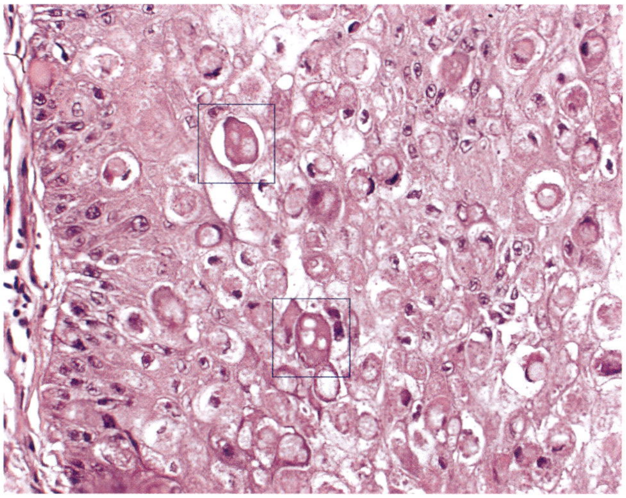

Figure 3.37: Bollinger's intracytoplasmatic bodies in a histological preparation of the *Stratum spinosum* of a pox-associated skin lesion from a Peregrine falcon. HE stain.

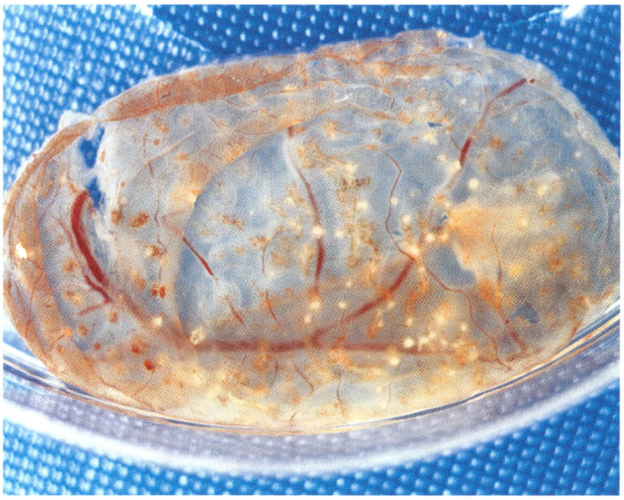

Figure 3.38: Pock-lesions on the chorio-allontoic membrane (CAM) five days after inoculation with a falconpox virus. An attenuated falconpox vaccine has been established by CVRL. This vaccine is annually administered to hundreds of hunting falcons prior to the hunting season.

3

Influenza

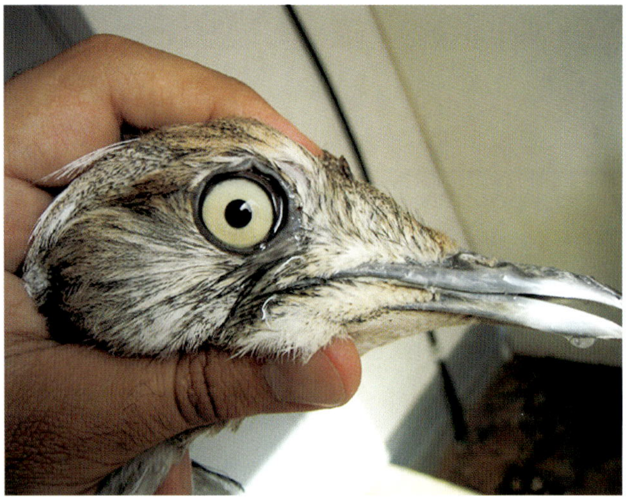

Figure 3.39: Discharge from eyes and nostrils of a Houbara Bustard (*Chlamydotis undulata*) with Influenza A infection. Hunting falcons contract their Influenza infection through their quarry.

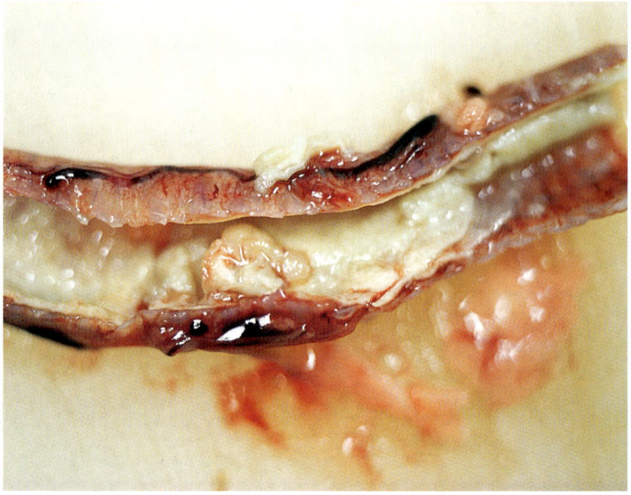

Figure 3.40: Severe tracheitis with pus production in a Houbara Bustard with Influenza A infection.

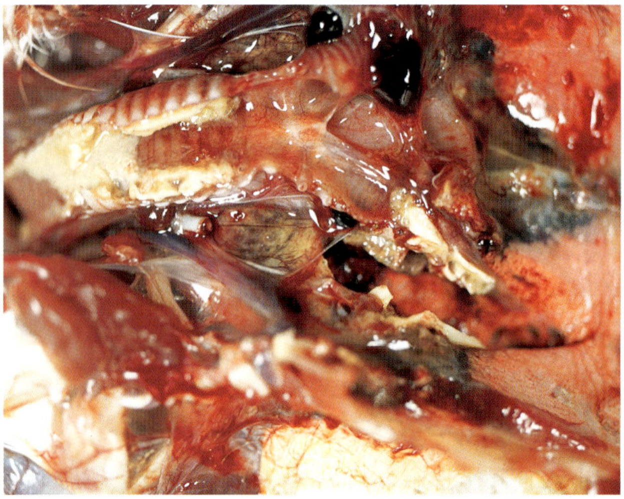

Figure 3.41: Pneumonia indicated by the dark-red areas in the lung as well as pus in the bronchi of a Houbara Bustard with influenza.

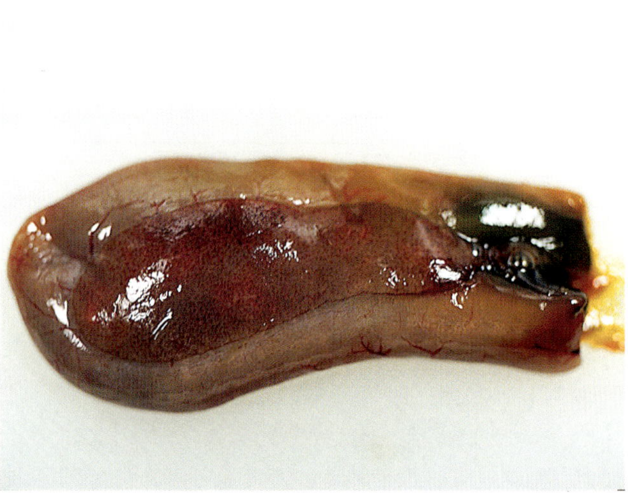

Figure 3.42: Pancreatitis in a Houbara Bustard caused by the influenza virus.

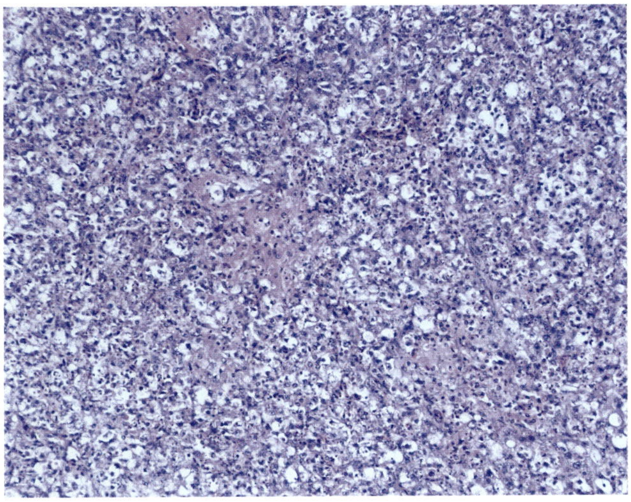

Figure 3.43: Pancreatitis in a Houbara Bustard: Atrophy of exocrine tissue with numerous small eosinophilic necrosis and marked diffuse infiltration with mononuclear cells. HE stain.

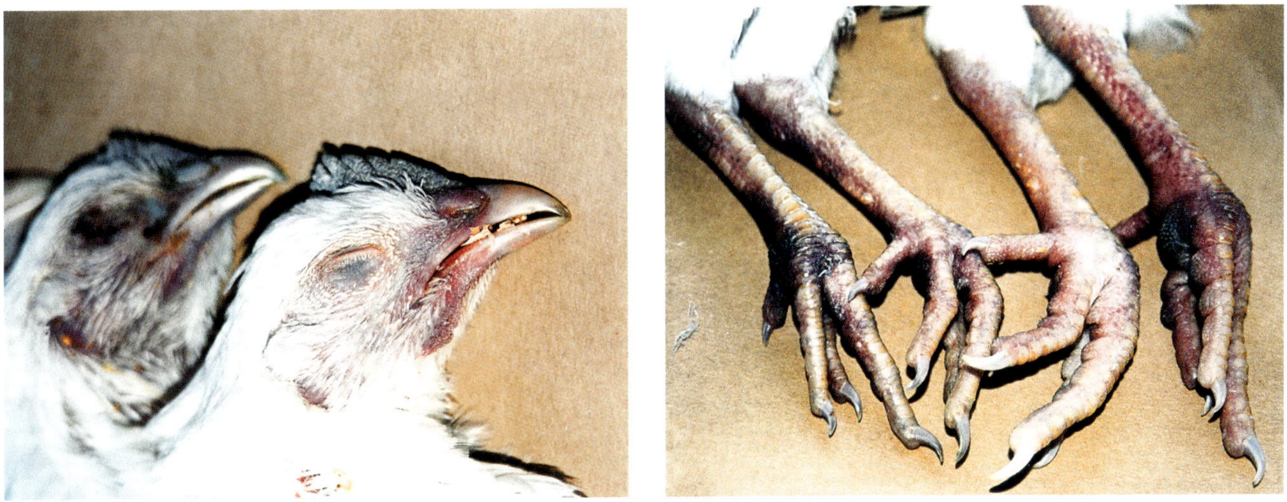

Figure 3.44 a, b: Acute cyanosis of wattles, combs and legs, 3 days after infection of 6-week-old chickens with a H7N3 Influenza A strain from a Peregrine falcon. Several cases have been described where avian flu type H5 and H9 lead to serious influenza in humans resulting fatalities.

Chapter 4

Bacterial Diseases

4

Hunting falcons may suffer from many different bacterial diseases, the lesions of which are shown on the next pages. Blood has been analysed from many of these cases, and the results are presented in Tables 4.1 and 4.2. The results show a slight decrease in haematology values and an increase in WBC and heterophils. Most of the biochemistry values are also elevated including total protein and globulin. In clostridial enterotoxaemia, however, the total WBC is often decreased, due to the destructive nature of the clostridial toxin on the blood producing centers, and some of the biochemistry parameters may be extremely high (CK, LDH, GGT, BA).

Heterophils are the most numerous of the granulocytes found in birds. An increase in circulating heterophils occurs in response to bacterial and fungal disease, tissue damage, stress, some metabolic diseases and myeloid leukaemias. In healthy falcons, the heterophils have a lobed, usually bi-lobed nucleus and cigar-shaped brick-red granules. Immaturity of heterophils is characterized by a decrease in number or absence of nuclear lobes (left shift). Heterophils and eosinophils can usually be differentiated by the appearance of their granules. However, in sick birds, the granules of heterophils may change in appearance and colour and give rise to problems in distinguishing between both cell types. Further problems may result when examining old blood samples and following inadequate fixation, both of which may result in loss of granulation or the development of toxic changes. However, toxic heterophils are often associated with severe bacterial infections as indicated in the following pictures. The changes in heterophils are occasionally reported using a scale, as explained on page 32.

Table 4.1: Haematology and biochemistry values of falcons suffering from bacterial diseases (except clostridiosis)

Parameters	SI Units	N	Mean ± SD Diseased Falcons	Reference Values
RBC	$x10^{12}/l$	83	▼ **3.04** ± 0.44	3.21 ± 0.30
HB	g/dl	83	▼ **13.33** ± 2.16	14.95 ± 1.39
HCT	l/l	83	▼ **0.40** ± 0.04	0.45 ± 0.04
MCV	fl	83	▼ **131.58** ± 6.69	139.85 ± 6.33
MCH	pg	83	▼ **43.85** ± 3.00	46.42 ± 2.55
WBC	$x10^{9}/l$	83	▲ **13.76** ± 2.91	9.64 ± 3.96
HETERO	%	84	▲ **65.04** ± 5.81	59.80 ± 12.87
LYMPHO	%	84	▼ **28.73** ± 4.60	34.67 ± 12.88
MONO	%	84	5.60 ± 2.15	4.46 ± 2.77
EOS	%	84	0.41	0.43
BASO	%	84	0.20	0.16
CK	U/L	59	▲ **946** ± 116	640 ± 210
LDH	U/L	41	▲ **1183** ± 130	1028 ± 385
ALT	U/L	41	▲ **101** ± 42	64.8 ± 28.9
AST	U/L	41	▲ **142** ± 57	93.1 ± 44.6
GGT	U/L	62	▲ **208** ± 74	14.0 ± 6.3
BUN	mmol/l	44	▲ **6.8** ± 2.8	4.7 ± 1.80
UA	µmol/l	57	441 ± 231	487 ± 267
BA	µmol/l	57	24.8 ± 6.4	22.3 ± 4.7
TP	g/l	35	▲ **32.0** ± 10.0	28.4 ± 6.5
ALB	g/l	25	10.7 ± 1.7	10.4 ± 1.9
GLOB	g/l	26	▲ **21.3** ± 8.3	18.0 ± 4.6
IRON	µmol/l	57	6.5 ± 1.2	6.1 ± 3.7
CA	mmol/l	57	2.1 ± 0.2	2.4 ± 0.3
PHOS	mmol/l	37	0.8 ± 0.2	0.7 ± 0.3

Haematological pictures of falcons with bacterial infections

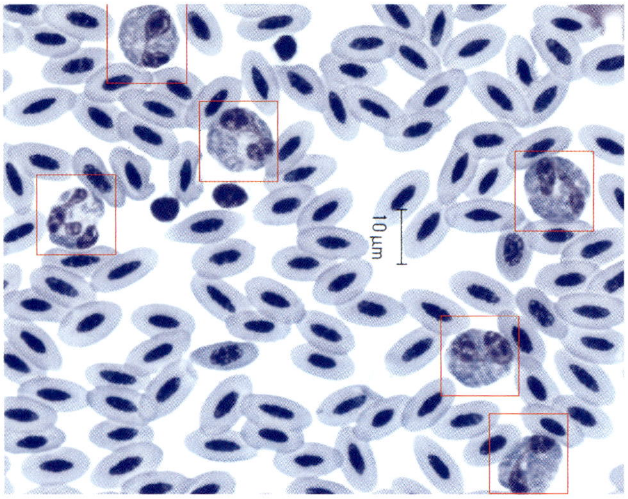

Figure 4.1: A Gyr hybrid with increased heterophils (heterophilia). Six heterophils and three thrombocytes are visible. This falcon suffered from chlamydophilosis.

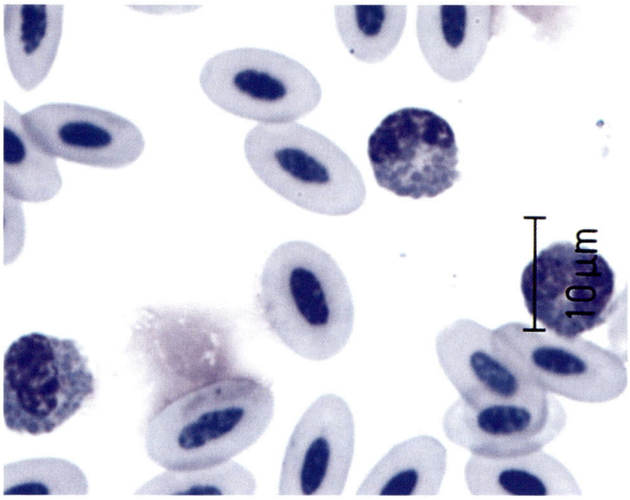

Figure 4.2: Three heterophils showing loss of lobulation and granulation as an indication of an inflammatory reaction. This Gyr hybrid had a salmonella infection.

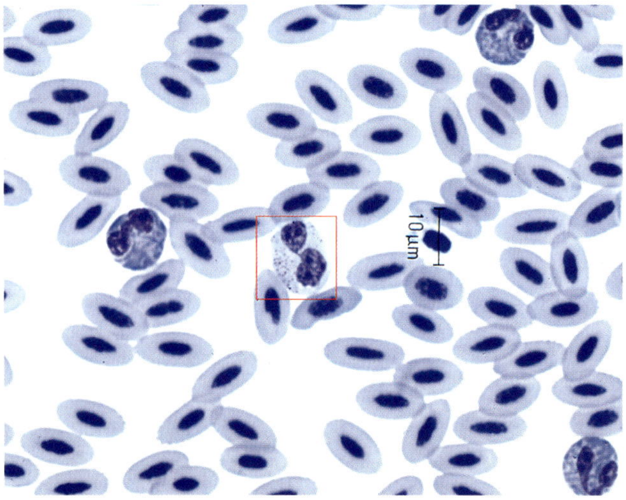

Figure 4.3: Three normal heterophils and one eosinophil (highlighted) of a Gyr hybrid with bumble foot.

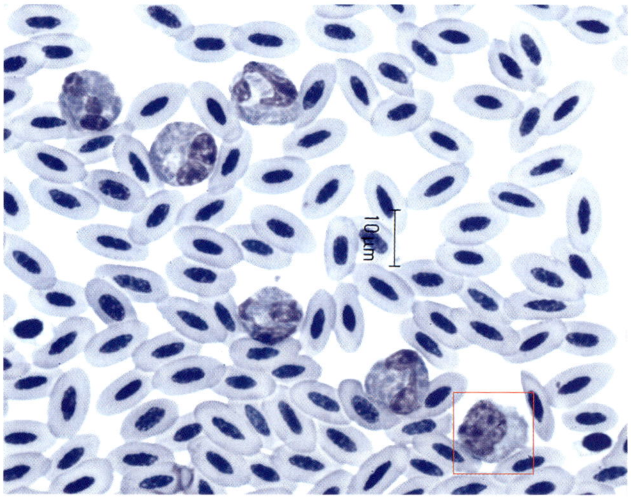

Figure 4.4: Five heterophils are visible (heterophilia) of which some show loss of granulation. This Gyr hybrid had bilateral bumblefoot (WBC 21 x 10^9/l, 78 % heterophils, 20 % lymphocytes, 2 % monocytes). One monocyte (highlighted) is also present.

4

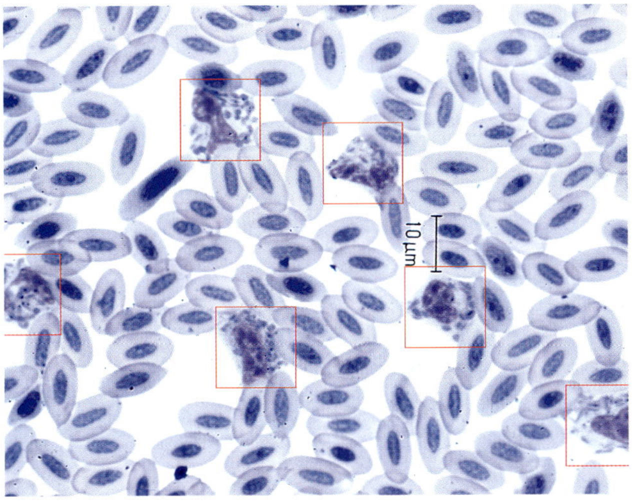

Figure 4.5: Six toxic heterophils (+4). This Saker falcon suffered from a bacterial airsacculitis.

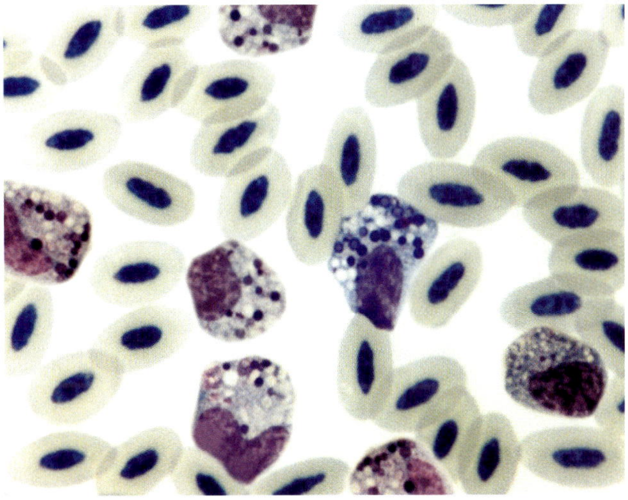

Figure 4.6: Seven toxic heterophils (+4) with loss of granulation and loss of lobulation from a Gyr hybrid with chronic bumblefoot (WBC 16.8 x 10^9/l, 82 % heterophils, 16 % lymphocytes, 2 % monocytes).

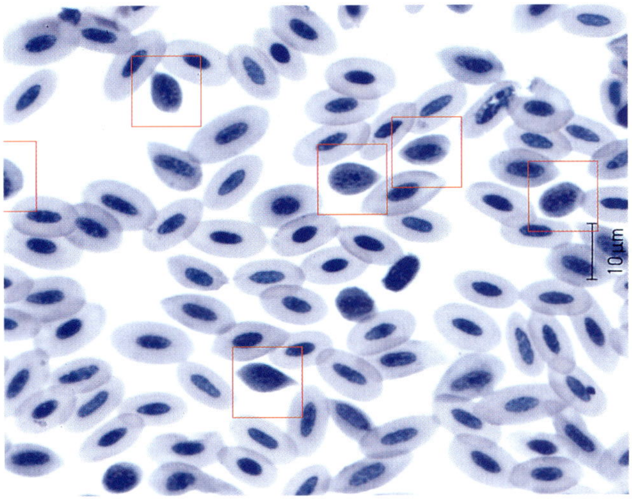

Figure 4.7: Several basophilic erythroblasts from a Gyr hybrid with regenerative anaemia associated with chronic airsacculitis. The red cells show poikilocytosis and anisocytosis.

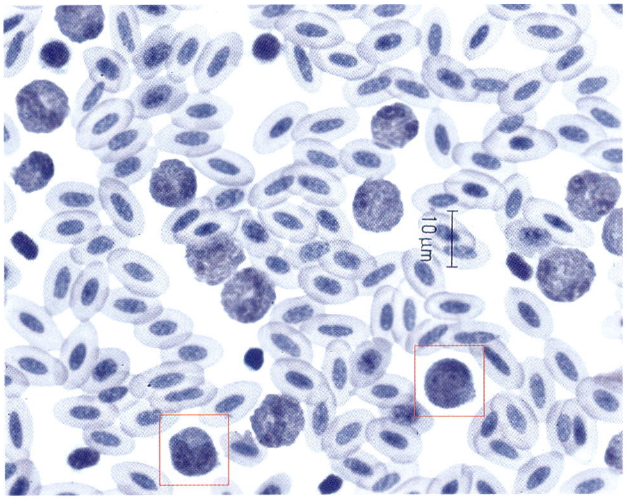

Figure 4.8: A Gyr hybrid with salmonellosis. Several heterophils, two monocytes (highlighted) and several thrombocytes are seen. The bird showed the following blood picture: WBC 19.6 x 10^9/l, 90 % heterophils, 4 % lymphocytes and 6 % monocytes.

Clostridium perfringens enterotoxaemia

Table 4.2: Haematology and biochemistry values of 15 falcons with clostridiosis

Parameters	SI Units	Mean ± SD Diseased Falcons	Reference Values
RBC	$x10^{12}/l$	▼ **2.19** ± 0.4	3.21 ± 0.30
HB	g/dl	▼ **10.70** ± 1.93	14.95 ± 1.39
HCT	l/l	▼ **0.32** ± 0.06	0.45 ± 0.04
MCV	fl	▲ **146.12** ± 7.34	139.85 ± 6.33
MCH	pg	▲ **48.86** ± 3.01	46.42 ± 2.55
WBC	$x10^{9}/l$	▼ **5.9** ± 2.0	9.64 ± 3.96
HETERO	%	▲ **64.0** ± 7.2	59.80 ± 12.87
LYMPHO	%	32.0 ± 4.1	34.84 ± 12.88
MONO	%	4.00 ± 2.00	4.46 ± 2.77
EOS	%	0.0	0.43
BASO	%	0.0	0.16
CK	U/L	▲ **1691** ± 410	640 ± 210
LDH	U/L	▲ **2140** ± 481	1028 ± 385
ALT	U/L	nd *	64.8 ± 28.9
AST	U/L	▲ **496** ± 96	93.1 ± 44.6
GGT	U/L	▲ **34.7** ± 6.4	14.0 ± 6.3
BUN	mmol/l	5.4 ± 1.3	4.7 ± 1.80
UA	µmol/l	nd	487 ± 267
BA	µmol/l	nd	22.3 ± 4.7
TP	g/l	26.3 ± 5.1	28.4 ± 6.5
ALB	g/l	10.1 ± 2.0	10.4 ± 1.9
GLOB	g/l	▼ **16.2** ± 3.1	18.0 ± 4.6
IRON	µmol/l	nd	6.1 ± 3.7
CA	mmol/l	nd	2.4 ± 0.3
PHOS	mmol/l	nd	0.7 ± 0.3

* nd = not done

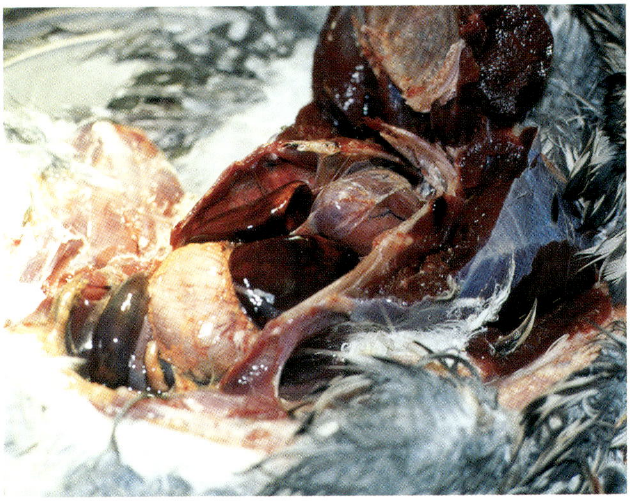

Figure 4.9: A Gyr falcon that died from *C. perfringens* enterotoxaemia. Swollen liver, pale heart and red intestines were observed during necropsy. Predisposing factors for the development of *C. perfringens* enterotoxaemia include concurrent diseases like aspergillosis, gout, parasitosis, adeno and reovirus-infections, chlamydophilosis, overexertion, dehydration, management problems and ingestion of contaminated meat. Clostridial hyperimmune antisera given intravenously may reduce falcon mortality.

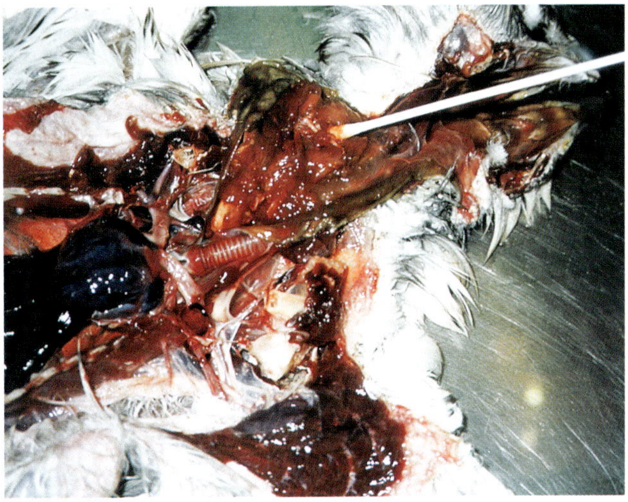

Figure 4.10: Gyr falcon which died from *C. perfringens* enteroxaemia caused by contaminated meat. This picture shows the opened crop with the meat from which a swab is taken. High numbers of *C. perfringens* organisms are frequently isolated from the crop.

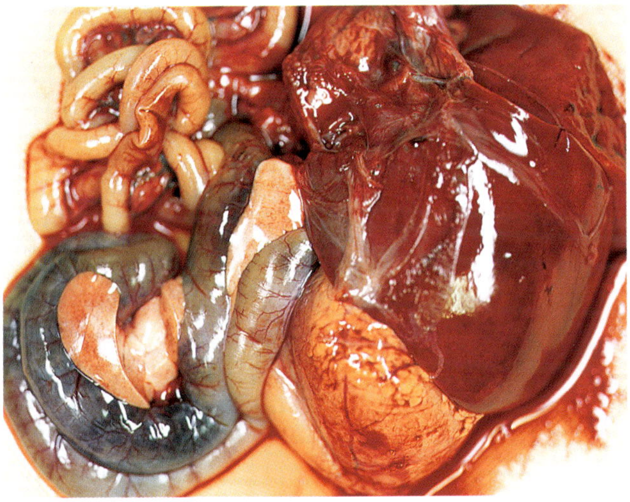

Figure 4.11: Haemorrhagic enteritis and enlarged liver in a falcon, which died from clostridial enterotoxaemia.

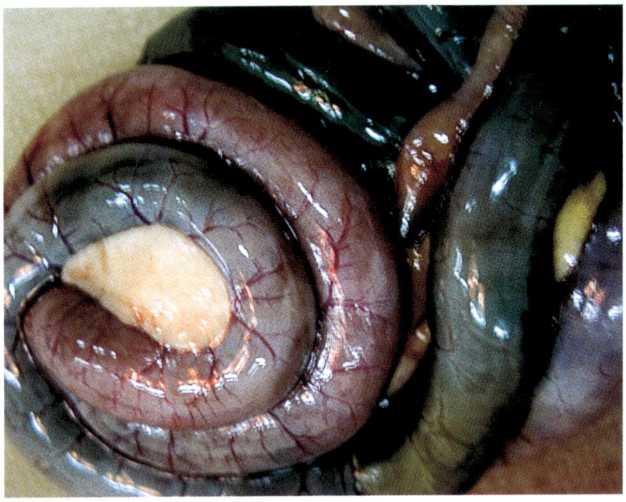

Figure 4.12: In severe clostridial enterotoxaemia cases, the intestines are filled with blood.

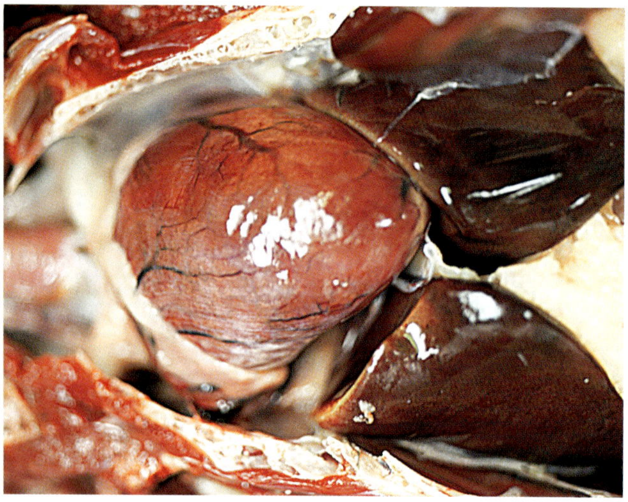

Figure 4.13: Pale heart muscle from a Gyr falcon with clostridial enterotoxaemia.

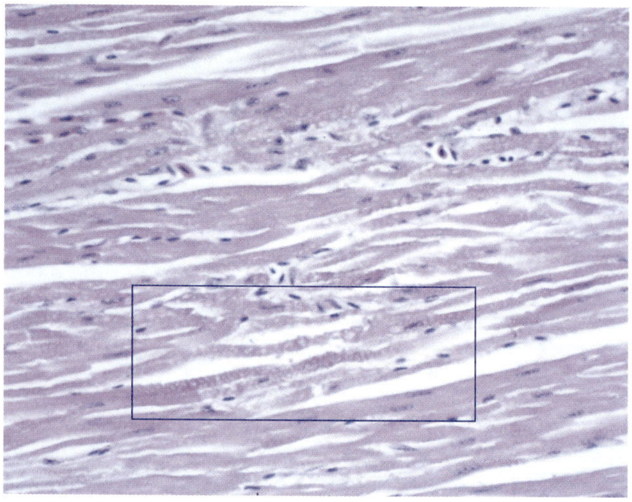

Figure 4.14: Heart of a Peregrine falcon showing acute degeneration of numerous muscle fibres. HE stain.

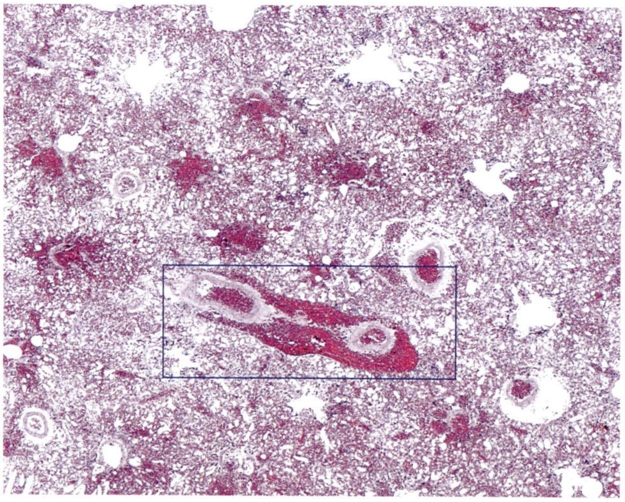

Figure 4.15: Lung with perivascular haemorrhages from a Gyr falcon, which died from clostridial enterotoxaemia. HE stain.

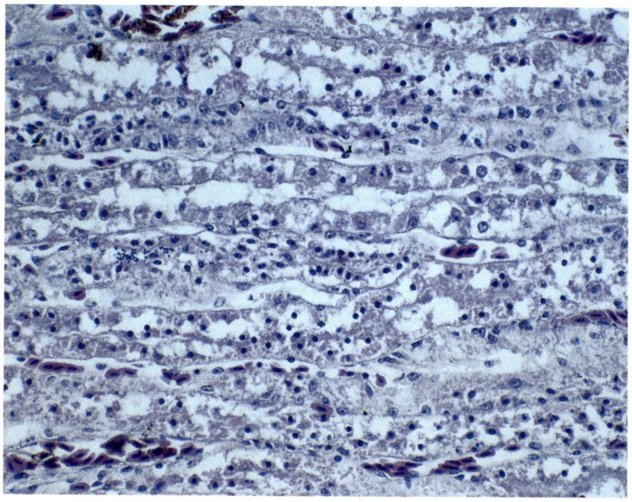

Figure 4.16: Kidney of a Gyr falcon with acute toxic degeneration of the distal renal tubuli caused by clostridial toxin. HE stain.

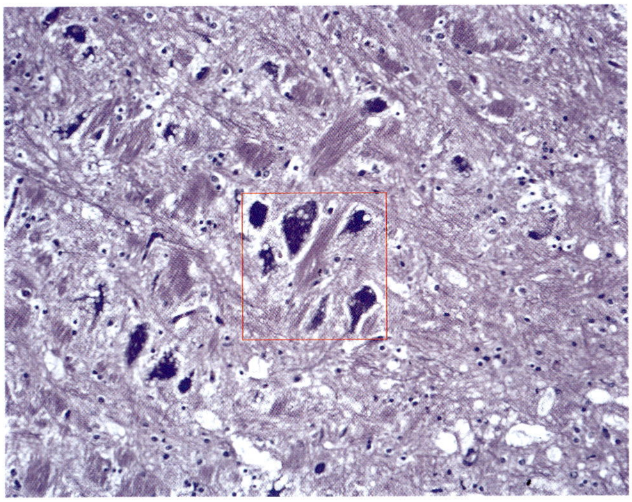

Figure 4.17: Brain of a Gyr falcon with focal symmetric encephalomalacia (FSE) that died from clostridial enterotoxaemia. Note the vacuolation of ganglion cells. HE stain.

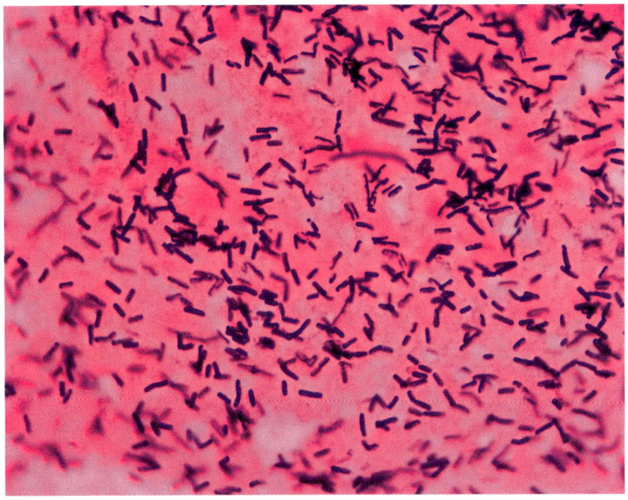

Figure 4.18: High numbers of Gram-positive rods from a direct smear of the intestinal mucosa of a Saker falcon which died from clostridial enterotoxaemia. Sixty percent of clinically normal falcons have been found to excrete *C. perfringens* organisms.

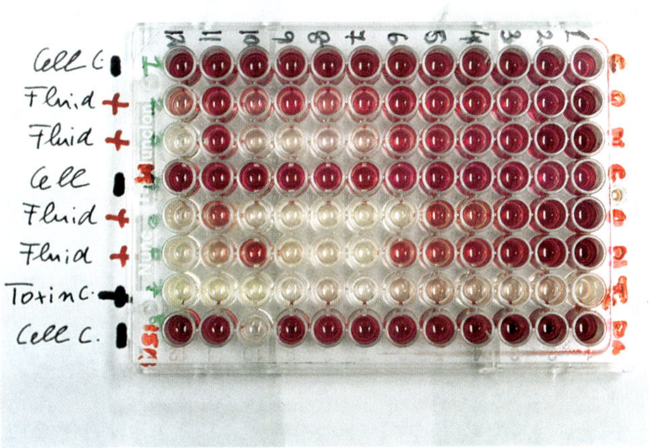

Figure 4.19: Colorimetric tetrazolium (MTT) cleavage test results on vervet monkey kidney cell cultures (Vero cells) indicating toxin in the intestinal fluid of dead falcons. The intestinal fluid is serially diluted in columns twelve to one. Light colour indicates presence of toxins.

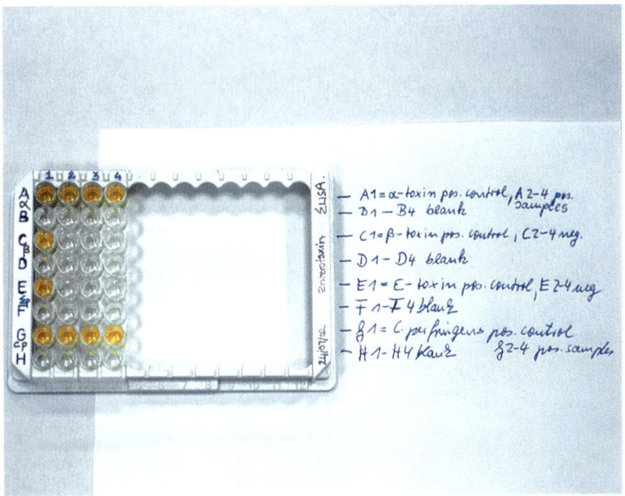

Figure 4.20: *C. perfringens* ELISA test results. MTT, ELISA and polymerase chain reaction (PCR) have replaced the mouse bioassay. This ELISA identifies 3 major *C. perfringens* toxins and the isolated strains: Samples two to four are positive for α-toxin (A 2–4) as well as for *C. perfringens* organisms (G 2–4).

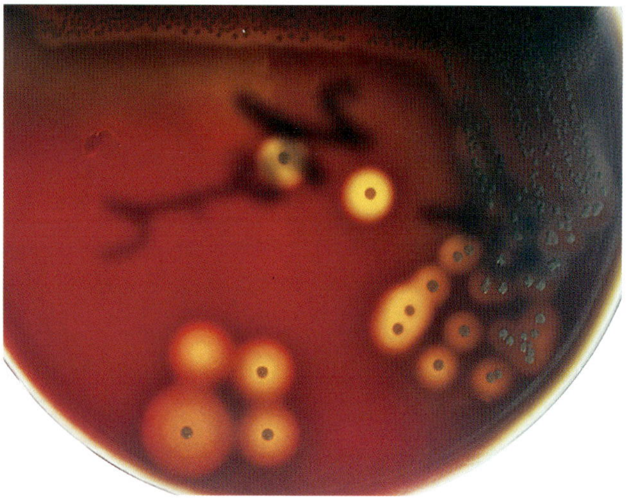

Figure 4.21: *C. perfringens* colonies on Zeissler agar. Note the typical double-zone haemolysis.

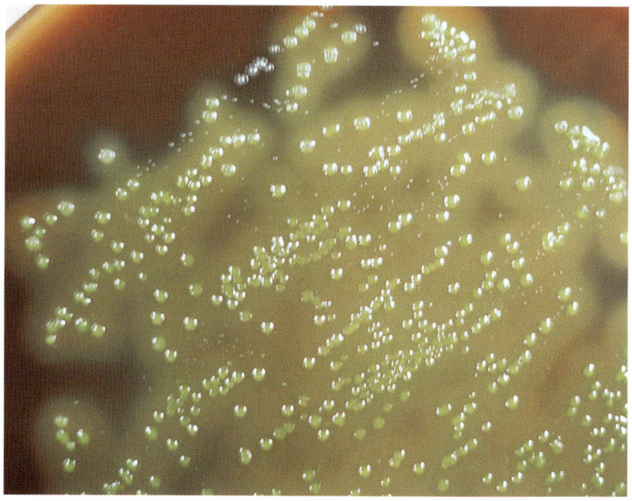

Figure 4.22: When the Zeissler agar plates are exposed to oxygen for several hours at room temperature, *C. perfringens* colonies produce a light green pigment

Chlamydophilosis

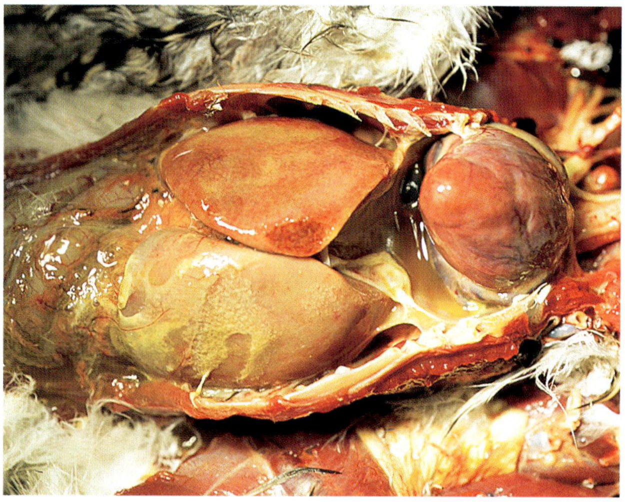

Figure 4.23: Peritonitis caused by *Chlamydophila* spp. in a Gyr hybrid. The disease in falcons is rare. However, pharyngeal swabs are often positive in the antigen-ELISA in falcons with no clinical signs. Frequently, the only history is »poor performance«. These are most probably subclinical cases. So far no serotyping of *Chlamydophila*-positive falcons have been performed.

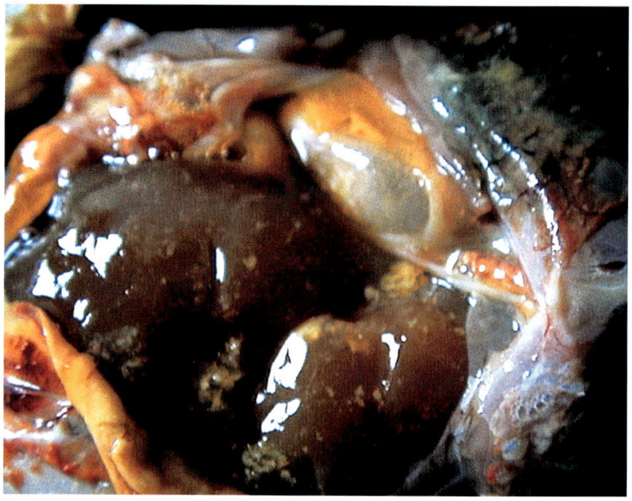

Figure 4.24: Hepatomegaly and serofibrinous serositis in a two-year-old Gyr falcon with marked gelatinous pericardial and perihepatic exudates

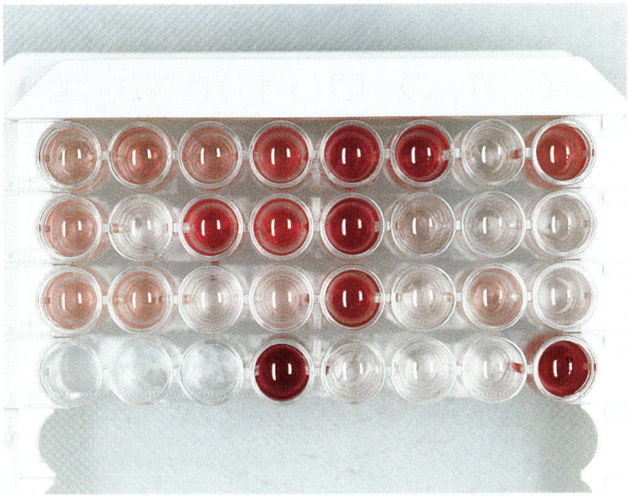

Figure 4.25: *Chlamydophila* antigen-ELISA. Wells which colour red are indicative of positive reactions. Swabs are taken from the pharynx, eyes or organ surfaces (mainly liver) and dispatched to the laboratory in a special transport medium.

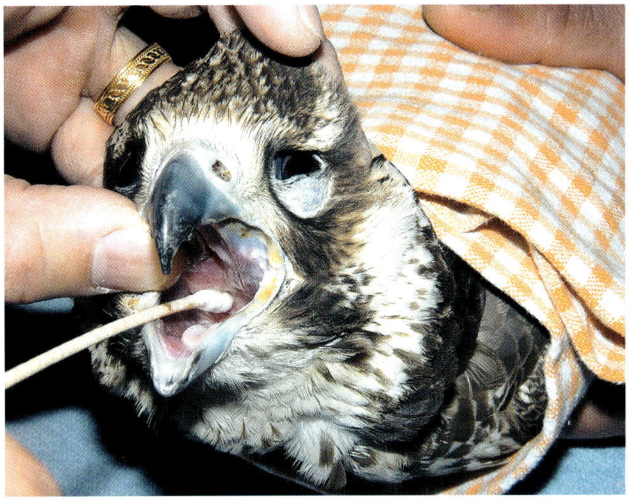

Figure 4.26: A swab is taken from the pharynx of a falcon for *Chlamydophila* diagnosis

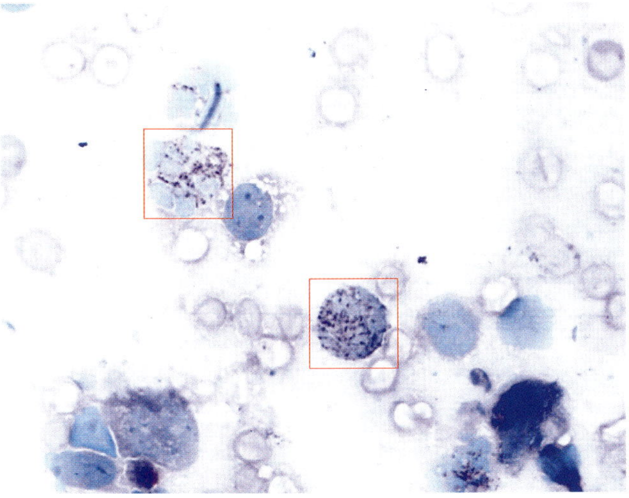

Figure 4.27: *Chlamydophila* inclusion bodies observed in the liver smear from a Saker falcon with chlamydophilosis. Gimenez stain.

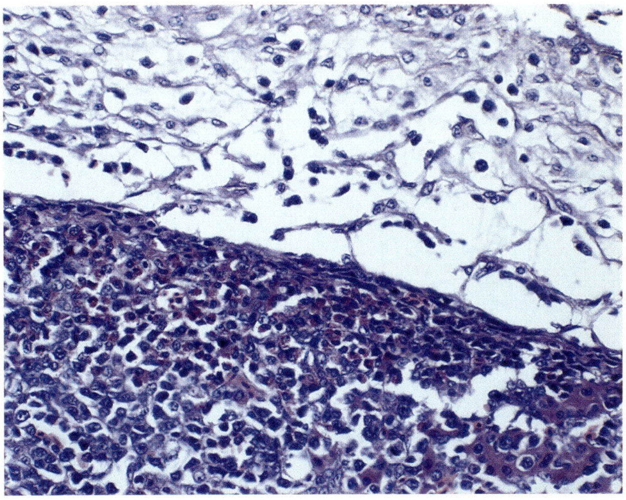

Figure 4.28: Lymphoplasmacytic hepatitis and perihepatitis of a Gyr hybrid with fibrin exudates on the serosa and diffuse mononuclear cell infiltration of subcapsular tissue caused by *Chlamydophila* spp. HE stain.

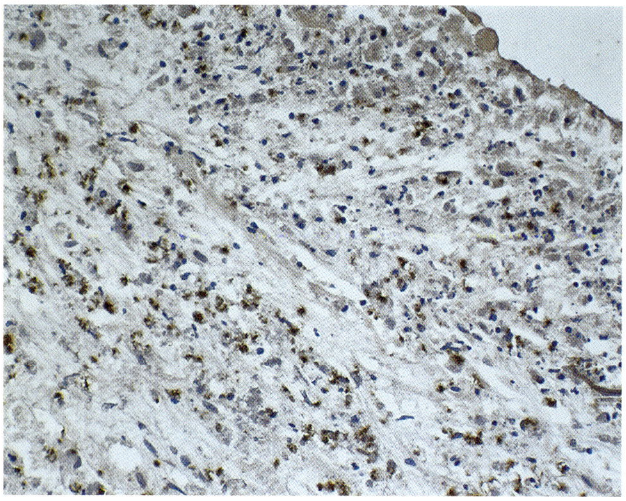

Figure 4.29: Immunohistochemistry of the same preparation of Figure 4.27: *Chlamydophila*-antigen positive particles are diffusely distributed in the fibrinous exudate (brownish staining).

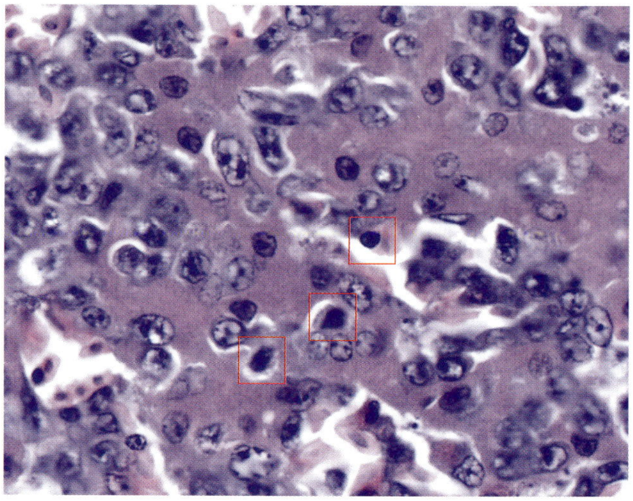

Figure 4.30: Lymphoplasmacytic hepatitis with numerous mononuclear cells in the sinusoids of a Saker falcon. The organisms suspected as *Chlamydophila* bacteria are seen in the center. HE stain.

Colisepticaemia

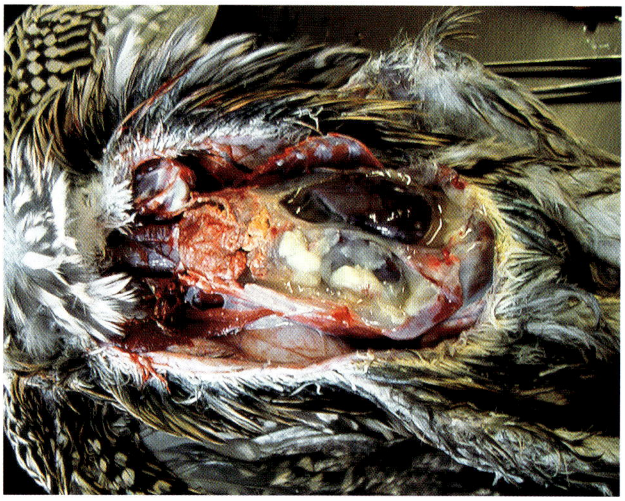

Figure 4.31: Massive subacute fibrinopurulent polyserositis with marked exudation of yellowish material on the pericardium and the peritoneum – a typical sign of bacterial induced serositis. Two-month-old Gyr x Peregrine hybrid.

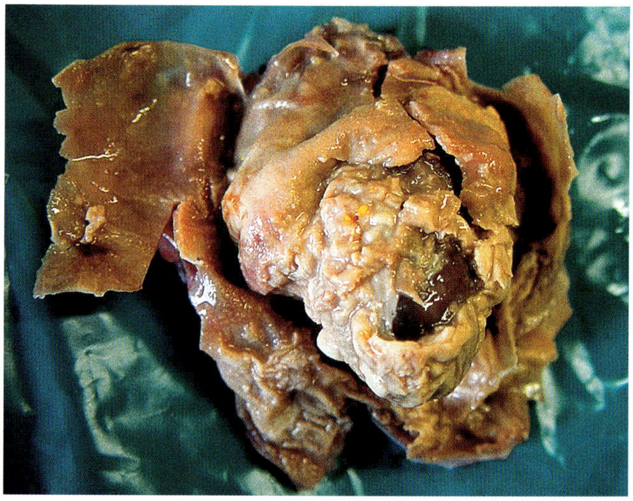

Figure 4.32: Severe subacute fibrinopurulent pericarditis with massive pericardial effusion in a Gyr x Peregrine caused by *E. coli.*

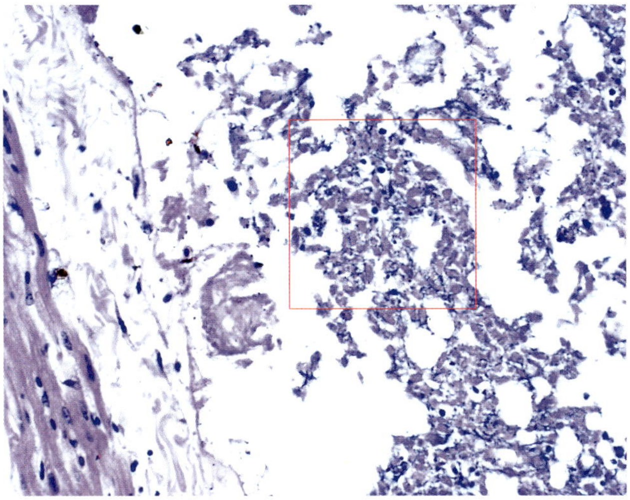

Figure 4.33: *E. coli* serofibrinous pericarditis in a Peregrine falcon. There are numerous bacteria visible in the debris of the pericardium. HE stain.

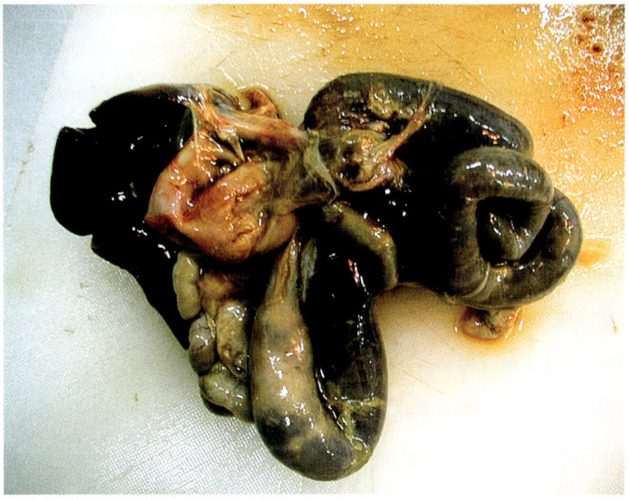

Figure 4.34: Mild fibrinous *E. coli* peritonitis in a one-year-old Gyr x Peregrine hybrid. Note the distention of the colon.

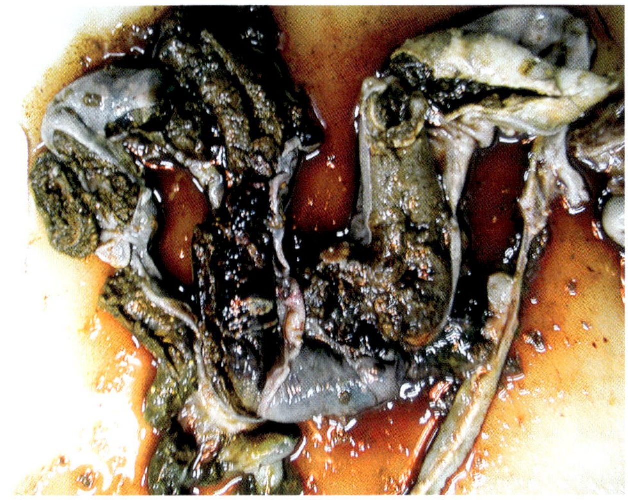

Figure 4.35: Opened colon of the same case as in Figure 4.33. Severe impaction with dry ingesta caused by *E. coli* induced peritonitis.

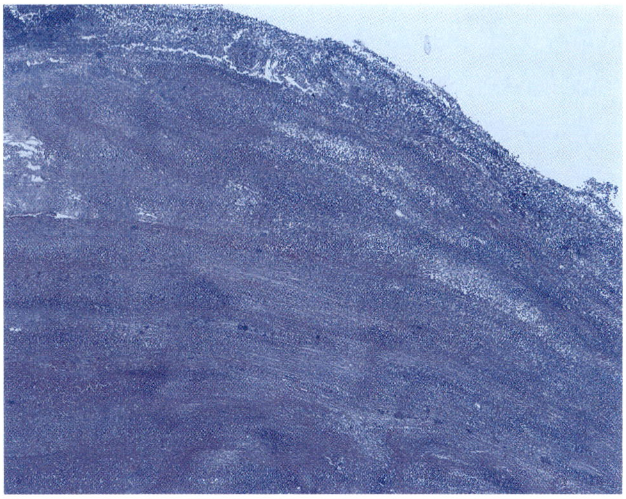

Figure 4.36: Histology of the same case as in Figure 4.34: Massive suppurative to necrotizing colitis caused by *E. coli*. Large necrotic mass in the colon lumen containing bacteria. Severe suppurative serositis. HE stain.

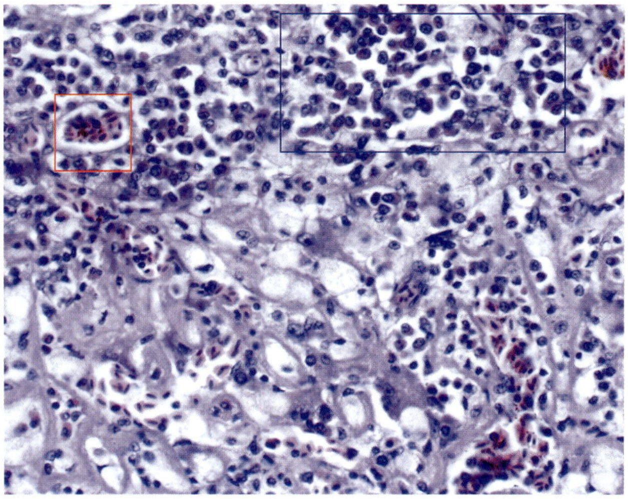

Figure 4.37: Suppurative hepatitis and perihepatitis of a Gyr hybrid caused by *E. coli* with marked infiltration with heterophils and macrophages (highlighted in blue) and some sinusoidal microthrombosis (highlighted in red). HE stain.

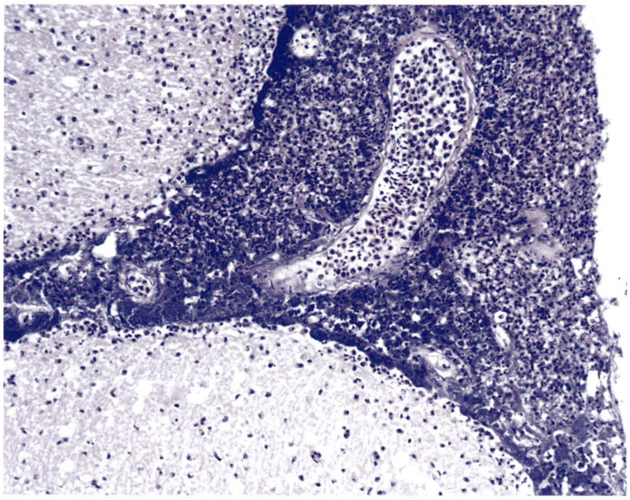

Figure 4.38: Severe suppurative meningitis of a Gyr falcon caused by *E. coli*. HE stain.

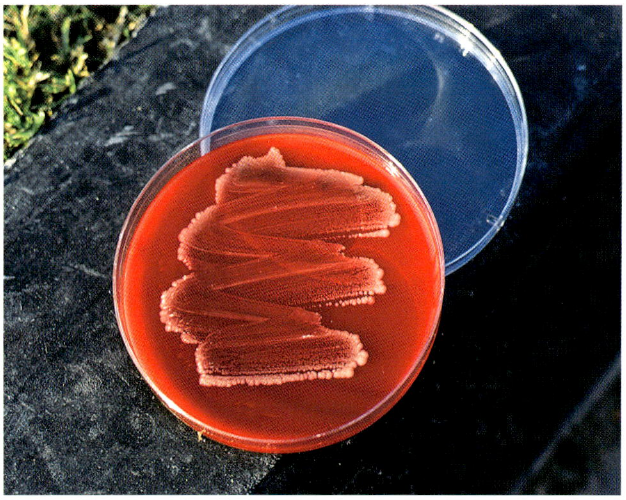

Figure 4.39: *E. coli* growth on blood agar isolated directly from the heart of a Peregrine. This is a heavy growth.

Pseudomonas septicaemia

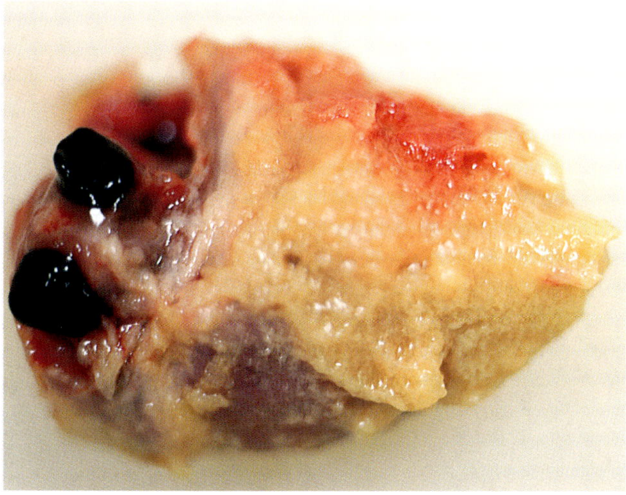

Figure 4.40: Massive fibrinopurulent pericarditis caused by *Pseudomonas aeruginosa* septicaemia in a Saker falcon.

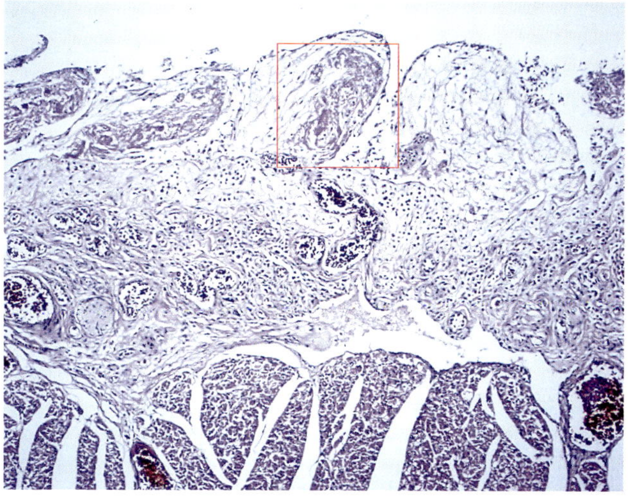

Figure 4.41: *P. aeruginosa* pericarditis: Fibrinopurulent pericarditis in a Gyr x Peregrine hybrid caused by *P. aeruginosa* showing bacteria in the exudate. HE stain.

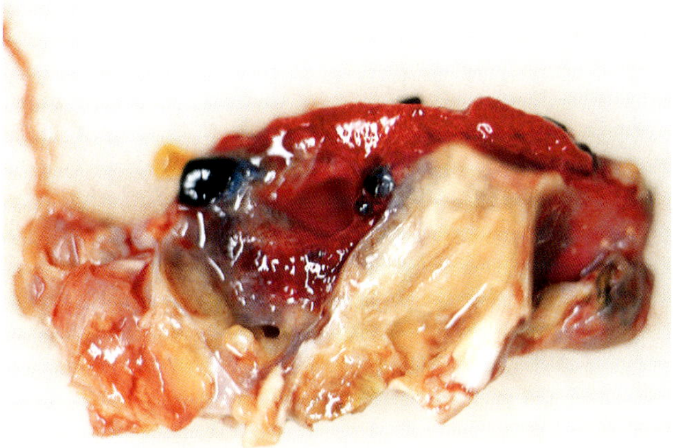

Figure 4.42: *P. aeruginosa* fibrinopurulent bronchitis and airsacculitis in a Peregrine falcon.

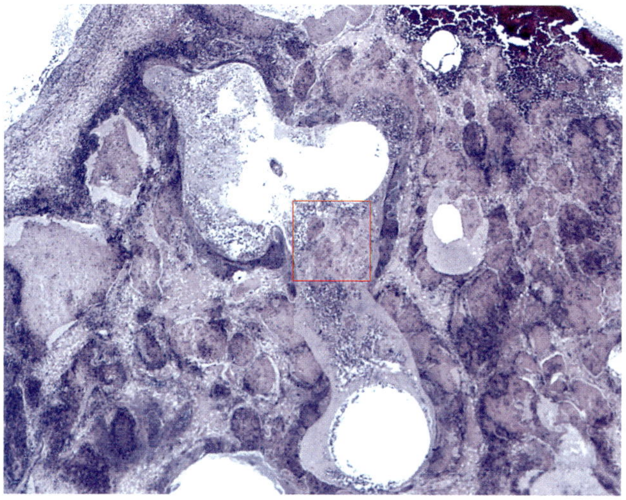

Figure 4.43: Fibrinopurulent to necrotizing pneumonia in a Gyr x Peregrine hybrid caused by *P. aeruginosa* showing bacteria in the exudate. HE stain

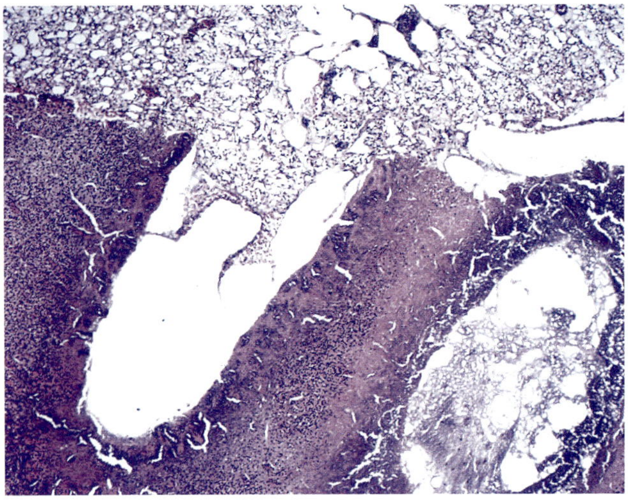

Figure 4.44: Massive exudative bronchitis caused by *P. aeruginosa* in a Peregrine falcon. Large bronchus completely filled with necrotic material and fibrin containing numerous bacteria. HE stain.

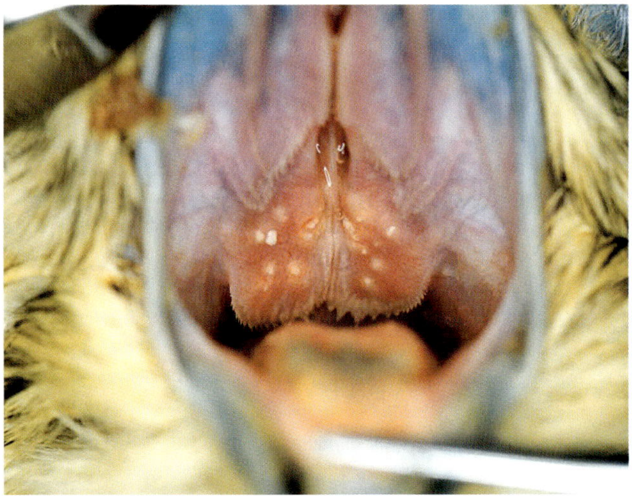

Figure 4.45: A Saker falcon (*Falco cherrug*) with stomatitis caused by *Pseudomonas aeruginosa.*

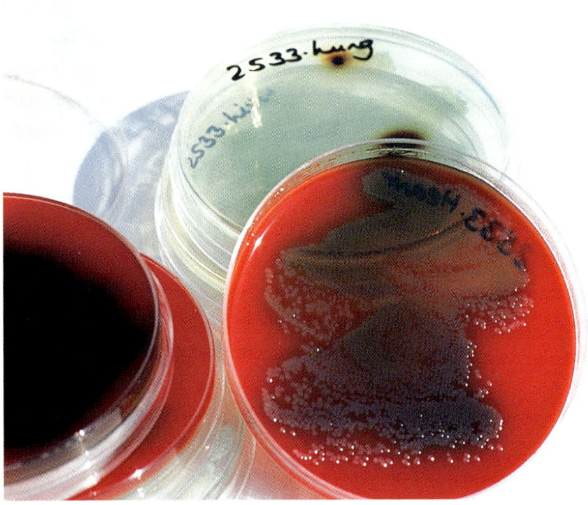

Figure 4.46: *P. aeruginosa* growth on blood and nutrient agar. The haemolysis on blood agar and the blue pigment on nutrient agar are typical for *P. aeruginosa*. *P. aeruginosa* is very resistant to many antibiotics and can grow at low temperatures.

Pasteurellosis

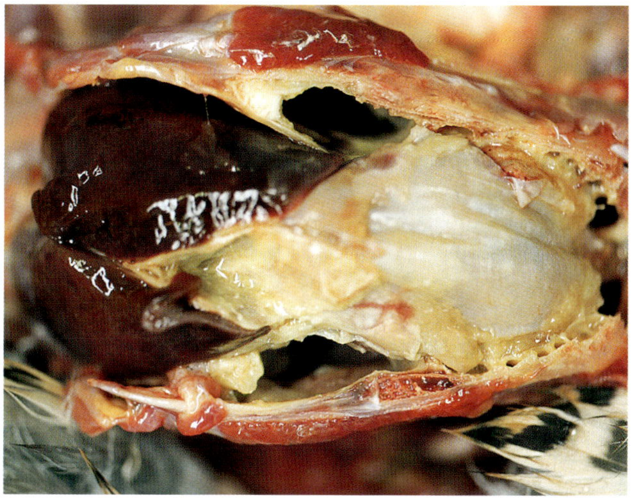

Figure 4.47: This Gyr falcon suffered from serofibrinous pericarditis caused by *Pasteurella multocida*. Pasteurellosis in falcons is caused by *Pasteurella multocida* or *Mannheimia haemolytica* which may cause pericarditis, perihepatitis, pneumonia, airsacculitis or serositis.

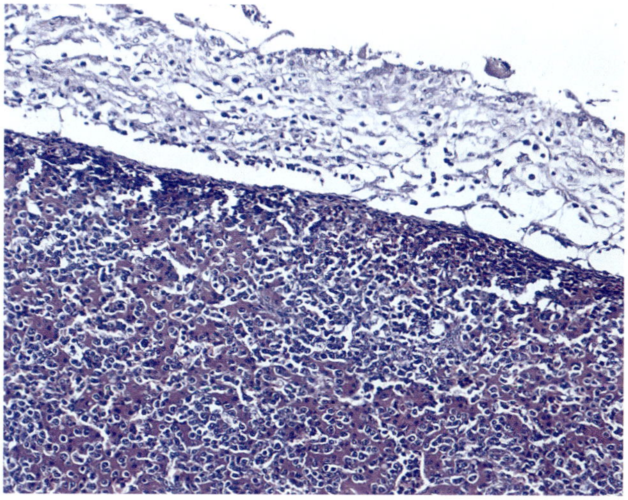

Figure 4.48: Pasteurellosis in falcon is rare and always linked to the ingestion of contaminated food. This picture shows the liver of a Saker falcon with marked serofibrinous perihepatitis with extensive acute inflammation. HE stain.

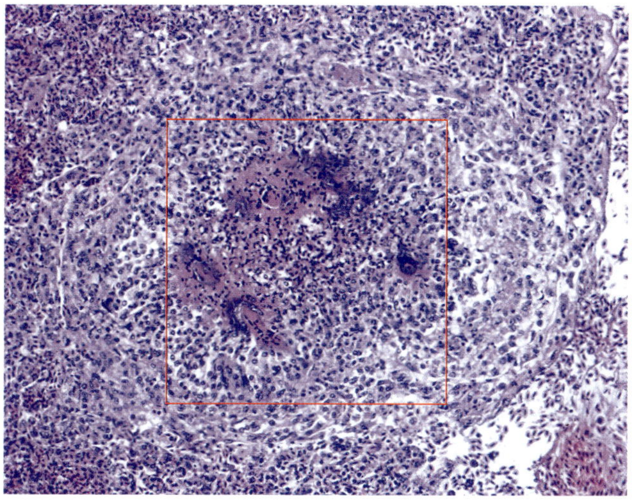

Figure 4.49: Pasteurellosis in a Gyr hybrid. Spleen with micro-abscesses containing numerous bacteria. Note the extensive inflammatory reaction around the bacteria. HE stain.

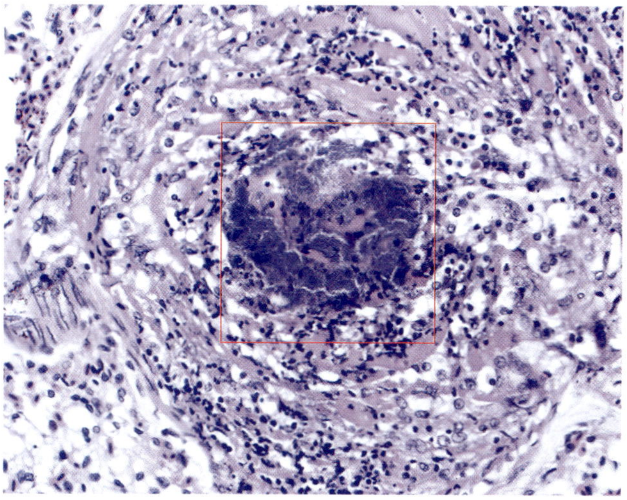

Figure 4.50: Pasteurellosis in a Peregrine falcon. Lung with an infectious thrombus in a vessel. HE stain.

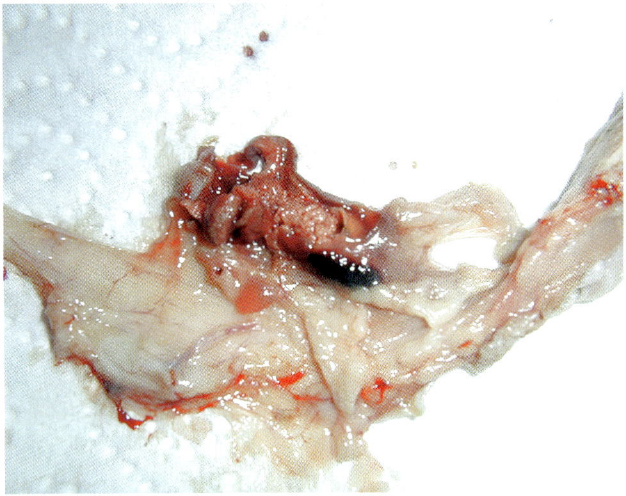

Figure 4.51: Crop infection caused by *Mannheimia haemolytica*. From many inflamed falcon crops, *Pasteurella* spp. is isolated, often in connection with *Staphylococcus aureus* and *Candida albicans*.

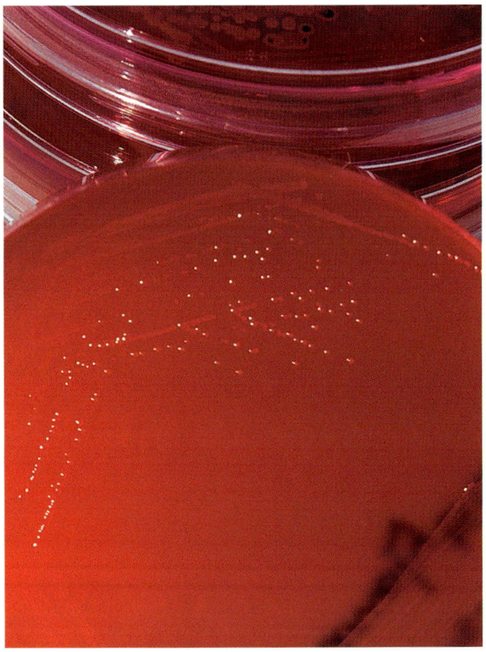

Figure 4.52: *Pasteurella* spp. colony growth on blood agar: Small transparent colonies.

Mycoplasmosis

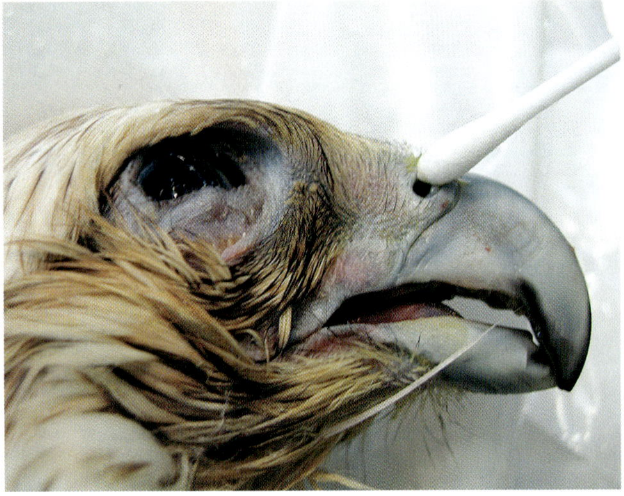

Figure 4.53: Taking a swab sample from a Saker falcon (*Falco cherrug*) affected with sinusitis.

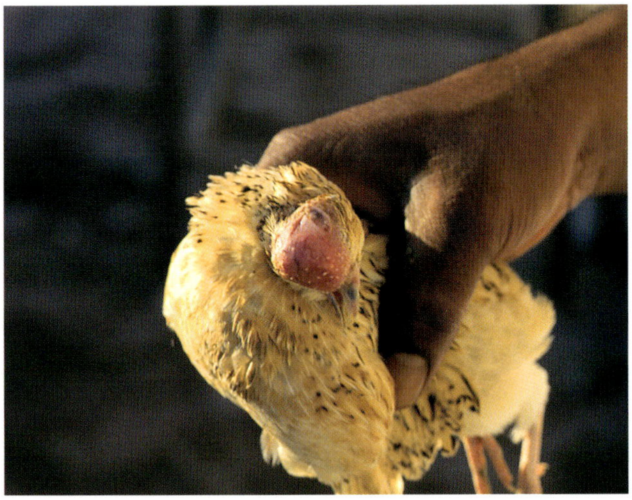

Figure 4.54: Quail with severe Chronic Respiratory Disease (CRD) caused by *Mycoplasma gallisepticum* associated with caseous sinusitis (owl head). Falcons may contract mycoplasmosis from ingesting diseased pigeons or quails.

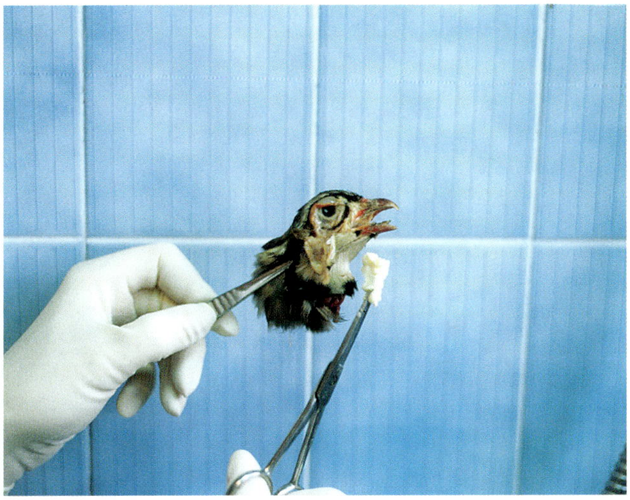

Figure 4.55: Arabian Red-legged Partridge (*Alectoris melanocephala*) with mycoplasmosis in which the infraorbital sinus is opened and the caseous material removed.

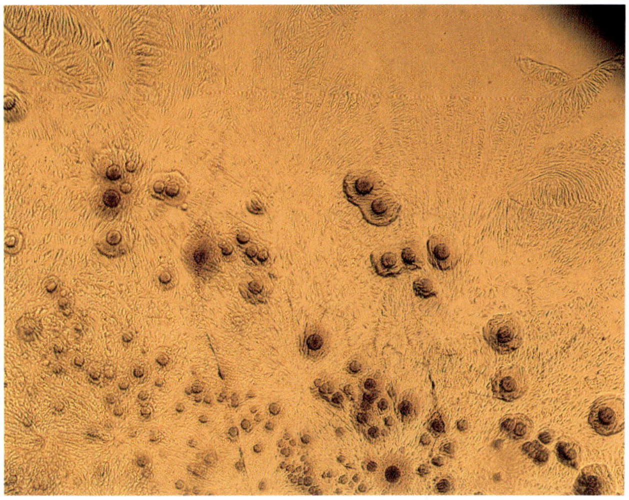

Figure 4.56: Typical »fried-egg« appearance of *Mycoplasma* spp. colonies on selective agar. Many different *Mycoplasma* species have been isolated from falcons, some of them cannot be serotyped.

Salmonellosis

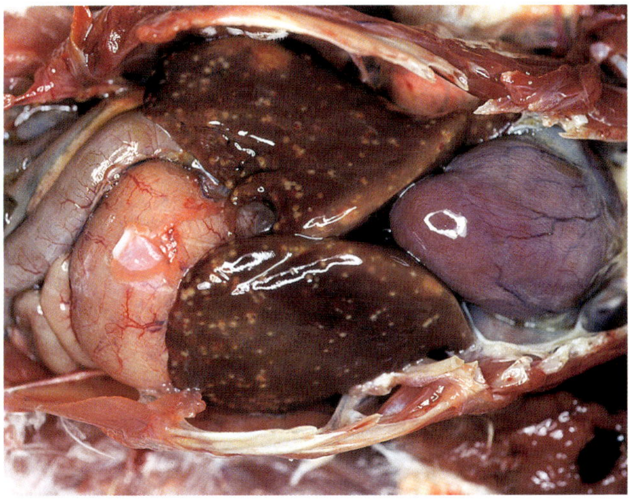

Figure 4.57: Miliar and supermiliar foci in an enlarged liver of a Gyr falcon with salmonellosis. This picture is very similar to inclusion body hepatitis (herpes). The enteric form of salmonellosis is rare in falcons.

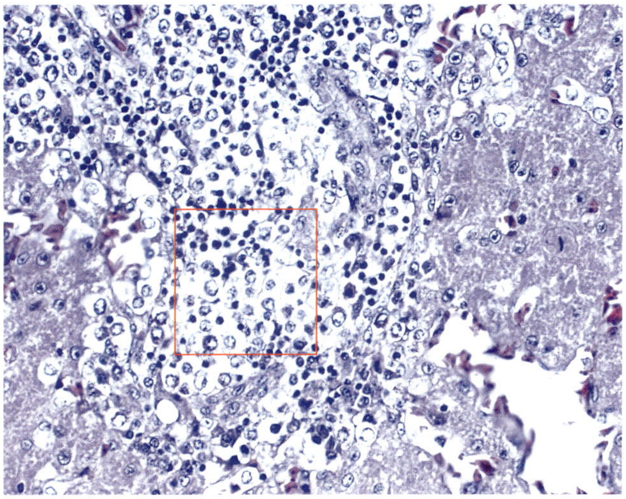

Figure 4.58: Focus of numerous apoptotic hepatocytes (focal acute necrosis) caused by salmonellosis in a Saker falcon. HE stain.

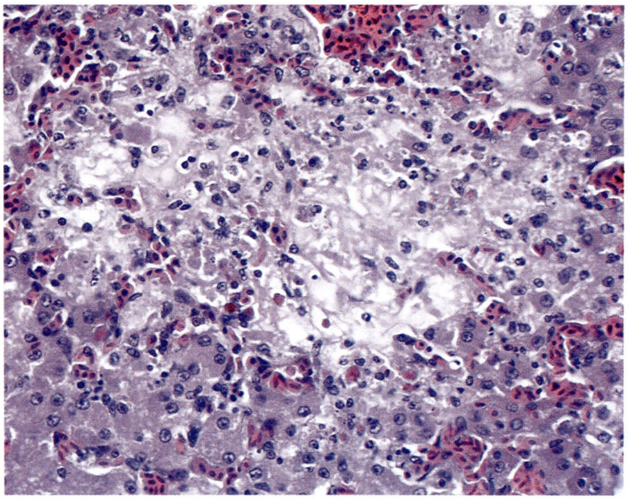

Figure 4.59: Liver: Necrotic focus with reactive infiltration (macrophages and heterophils) caused by salmonellosis in a Gyr falcon. HE stain.

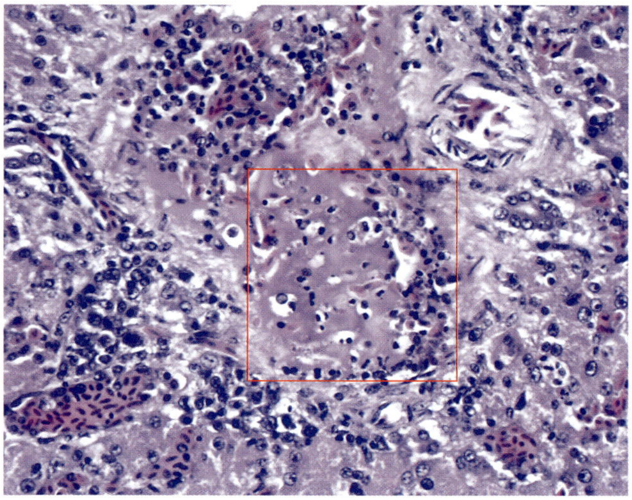

Figure 4.60: Thrombosed capillary causing necrobiosis of hepatic tissue. HE stain.

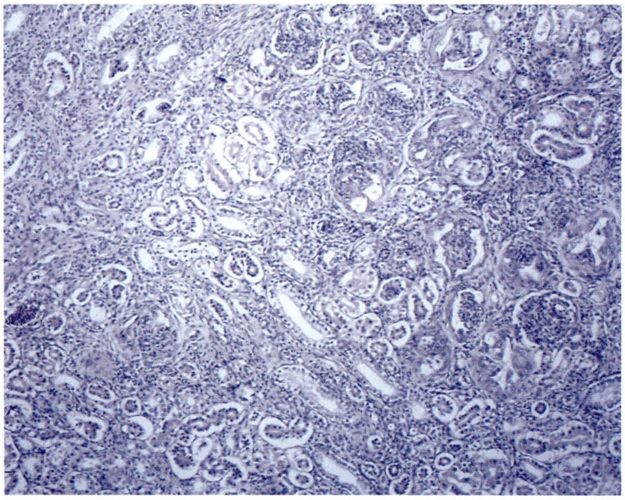

Figure 4.61: Subacute interstitial nephritis with tubular loss and mononuclear cell interstitial infiltrate caused by *Salmonella* spp. in a Gyr falcon. HE stain.

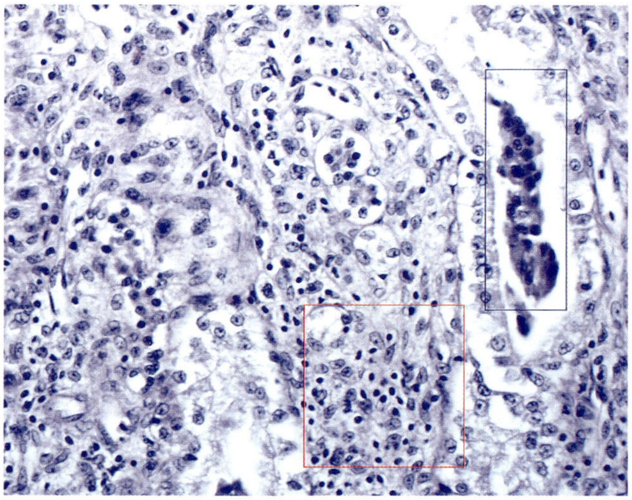

Figure 4.62: Detail of Figure 4.61: Diffuse mononuclear interstitial infiltrate and cellular debris in renal tubular lumen (highlighted in blue). HE stain.

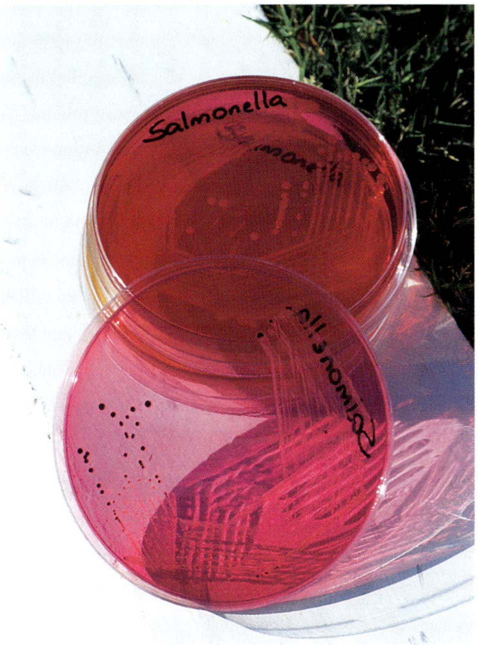

Figure 4.63: The colony growth of *Salmonella* spp. on different selective agars. Many different *Salmonella* serovars have been isolated from diseased and healthy falcons.

Tetanus

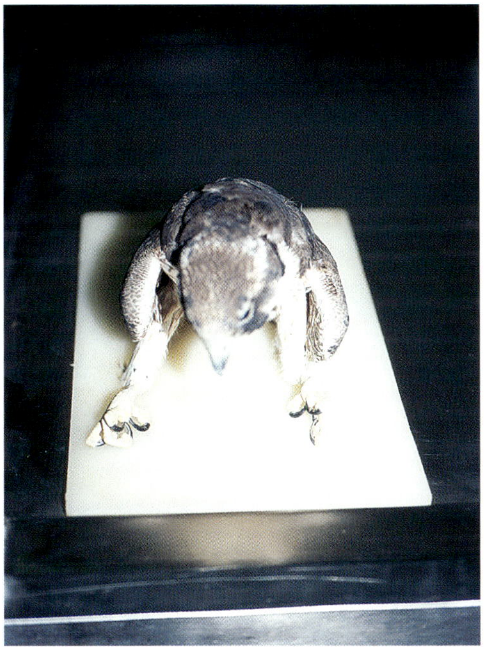

Figure 4.64: Tetanus in a Lanner falcon, exhibiting severe muscle spasms, resulting in extensor rigidity. Birds seem to be less sensitive to *Clostridium tetani* and consequently tetanus in birds is rare. However, a few cases are known.

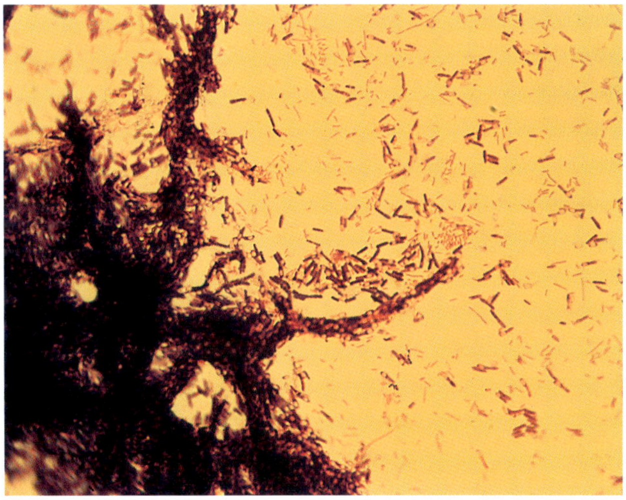

Figure 4.65: Characteristic »drumstick« sporing forms of *Clostridium tetani* observed in necrotic tissue removed from the right thigh wound of the Lanner falcon.

4

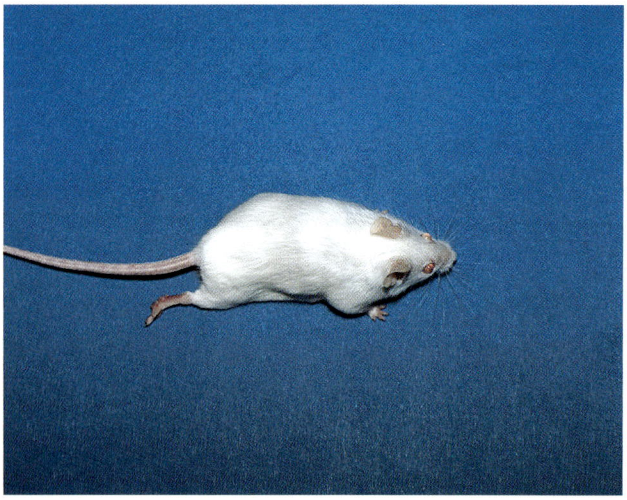

Figure 4.66: »Tetanic spasm« of the hind leg of a mouse inoculated with 0.1 ml of *Clostridium tetani* filtrate from thioglycollate broth.

Tuberculosis

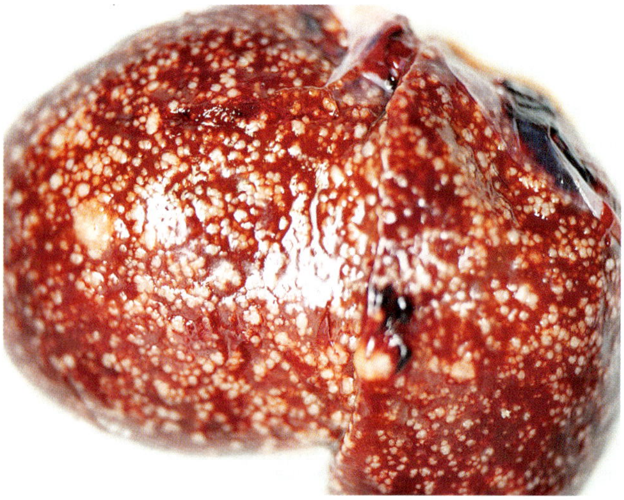

Figure 4.67: Generalised form of avian tuberculosis with involvement of the visceral organs in a Saker falcon (all following pictures are from the same Saker falcon). Enlarged spleen with numerous miliar whitish nodules (tuberculous granulomas). In all cases *Mycobacterium avium* was identified by PCR.

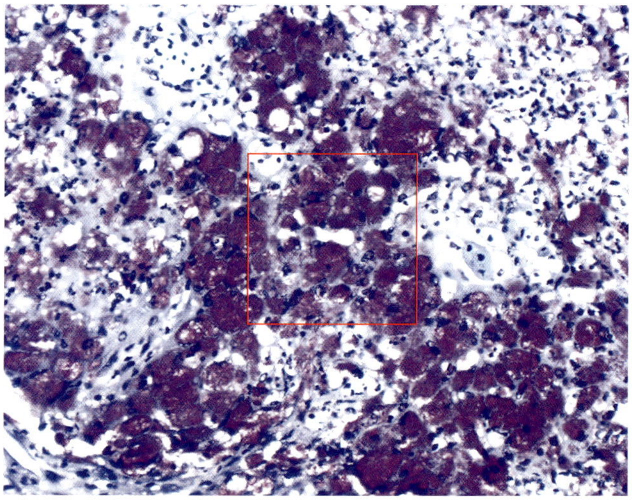

Figure 4.68: Tuberculous granuloma with numerous macrophages filled with acid-fast rods. Ziehl-Neelsen stain.

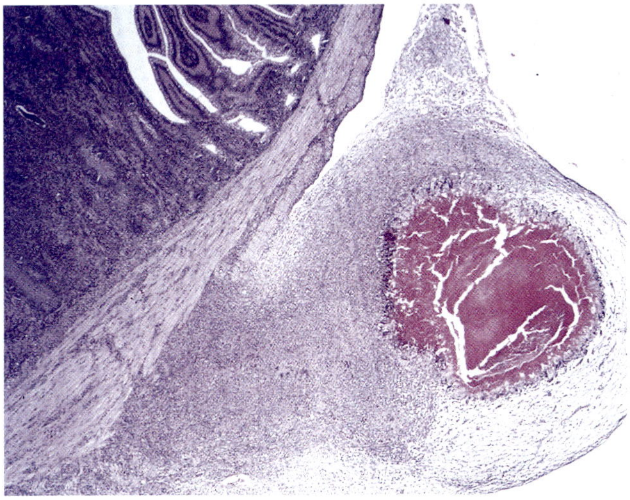

Figure 4.69: Avian tuberculosis often involves the intestine as seen in this case: Central necrotic granuloma on the serosa and proliferative enteritis. The enteric lesions are often considered to be the primary lesions. HE stain.

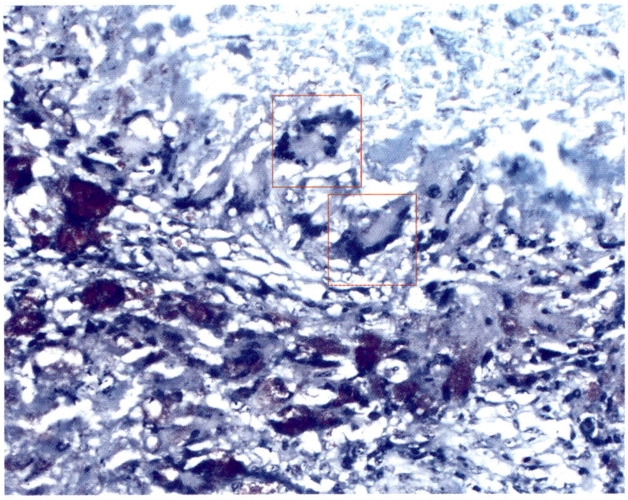

Figure 4.70: Higher magnification of Figure 4.69: Numerous macrophages surround the necrotic focus and some multinucleated giant cells (Langerhans-giant cells, highlighted) are also visible. Ziehl-Neelsen stain.

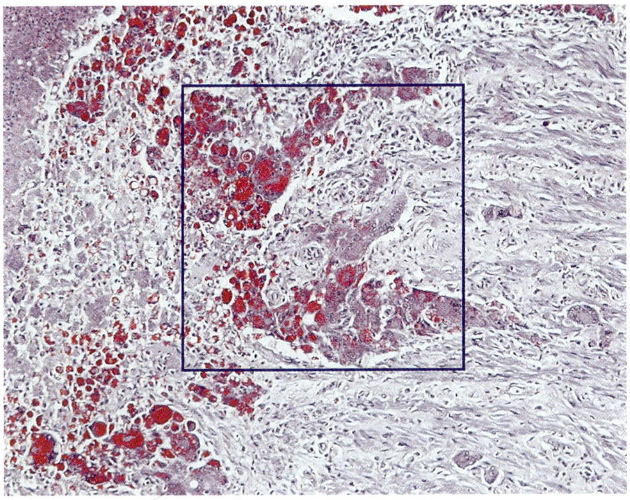

Figure 4.71 a: Proliferative enteritis with numerous macrophages filled with acid-fast rods. Ziehl-Neelsen stain.

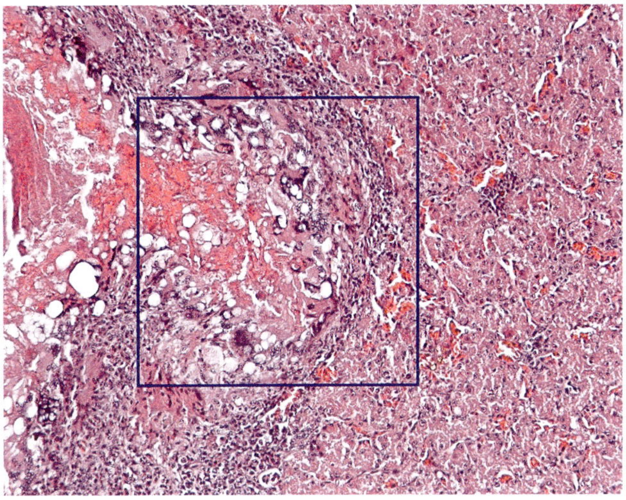

Figure 4.71 b: Tuberculosis of the liver in a Saker falcon showing a tuberculous granuloma with numerous Langerhans-giant cells. HE stain.

Figure 4.71 c
▶▶

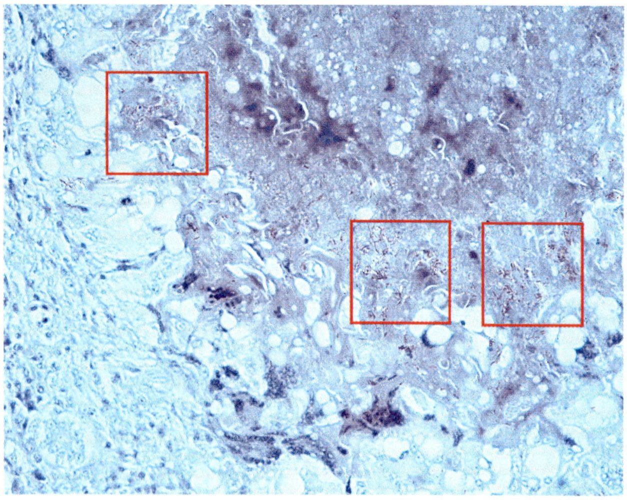

Figure 4.71 c: Higher magnification of Figure 4.71 b showing numerous acid fast rods. Ziehl-Neelsen stain.

Chapter 5

Fungal Diseases

Aspergillosis

Other fungal diseases

Candidiasis

Aspergillosis, caused by infection with *Aspergillus (A.) fumigatus* and less commonly by other *Aspergillus* species, is a debilitating very common respiratory disease of falcons in the Middle East. *A. fumigatus* is a ubiquitous saprophyte and opportunistic fungal pathogen, and inhalation of airborne conidia is the principle mode of infection. The pathogenesis of aspergillosis is highly complicated, especially as most of the strains are toxin producers. However, the toxins that are produced by *A. fumigatus* have not been thoroughly investigated. During our investigations on raptor aspergillosis we observed that over 95 % of fungal isolates from aspergillosis lesions were *A. fumigatus* of which more than 50 % were toxin producers. It is known that some of the toxins suppress the immune system of the falcon (e. g. Gliotoxin), predisposing to the development of other conditions such as bumblefoot or clostridial enterotoxaemia.

Candida albicans is commonly associated with disease in animals. Cell-wall glycoproteins have an endotoxin-like activity. In falcons mucous membranes and the foot may be involved. It can cause severe crop infection resulting in a thickened wall covered with pseudomembranous, yellowish-grey necrotic material similar to trichomonosis. *Candida albicans* may also be involved in the development of bumblefoot. Prolonged antibiotic therapy and malnutrition can initiate the infection.

Other fungal infections which are of less importance are caused by *Aspergillus flavus*, *Aspergillus nidulans* and *Blastomyces* spp.

Haematology and biochemistry parameters (Table 5.1) show a slight anaemia, increased WBC count, whereas blood chemistry changes are consistent with liver and kidney involvement as well as increased TP and mineral concentrations.

Table 5.1: Haematology and biochemistry values of falcons suffering from aspergillosis

Parameters	SI Units	N	Mean ± SD Diseased Falcons	Reference Values
RBC	$x10^{12}/l$	41	▼ **3.07** ± 0.45	3.21 ± 0.30
HB	g/dl	41	14.33 ± 1.98	14.95 ± 1.39
HCT	l/l	41	▼ **0.43** ± 0.06	0.45 ± 0.04
MCV	fl	41	140.07 ± 7.01	139.85 ± 6.33
MCH	pg	41	46.68 ± 2.54	46.42 ± 2.55
WBC	$x10^{9}/l$	41	▲ **13.97** ± 2.59	9.64 ± 3.96
HETERO	%	41	60.51 ± 18.38	59.80 ± 12.87
LYMPHO	%	41	33.85 ± 17.84	34.84 ± 12.88
MONO	%	41	5.43 ± 2.45	4.46 ± 2.77
EOS	%	41	0.05	0.43
BASO	%	41	0.05	0.16
CK	U/L	41	▲ **943** ± 114	640 ± 210
LDH	U/L	38	981 ± 364	1028 ± 385
ALT	U/L	38	▲ **570** ± 212	64.8 ± 28.9
AST	U/L	41	▲ **163.6** ± 32.1	93.1 ± 44.6
GGT	U/L	38	▲ **19.4** ± 7.1	14.0 ± 6.3
BUN	mmol/l	49	▲ **6.3** ± 1.9	4.7 ± 1.8
UA	µmol/l	49	▲ **563** ± 230	487 ± 267
BA	µmol/l	61	▲ **72.7** ± 5.9	22.3 ± 4.7
TP	g/l	41	▲ **33.5** ± 7.2	28.4 ± 6.5
ALB	g/l	41	10.5 ± 1.6	10.4 ± 1.9
GLOB	g/l	41	▲ **23.0** ± 6.9	18.0 ± 4.6
IRON	µmol/l	50	▲ **10.6** ± 1.4	6.1 ± 3.7
CA	mmol/l	38	▲ **2.8** ± 0.4	2.4 ± 0.3
PHOS	mmol/l	41	▲ **1.1** ± 0.6	0.7 ± 0.3

5

Haematology pictures of aspergillosis

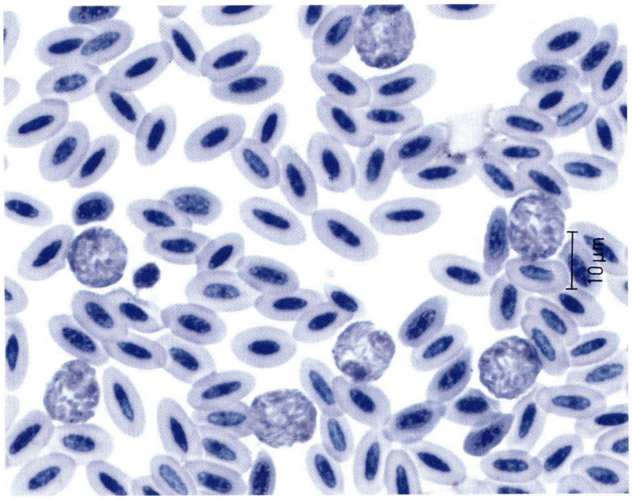

Figure 5.1: Heterophilia in a Gyr falcon with aspergillosis (WBC 16.9 x 10^9/l, 86 % heterophils, 10 % lymphocytes, 4 % monocytes). Seven heterophils are visible.

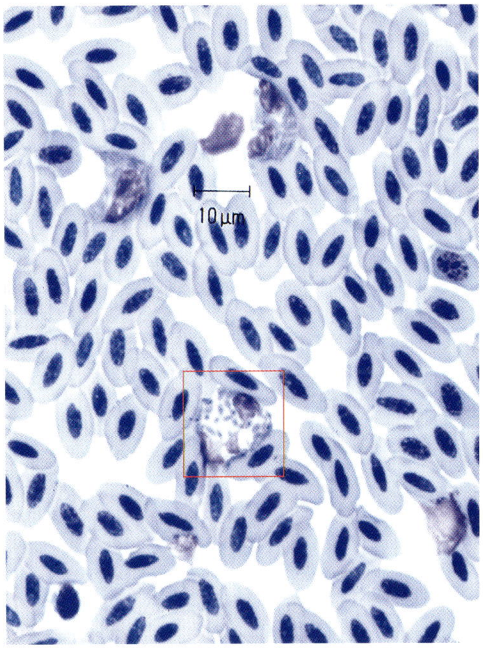

Figure 5.2: Chronic aspergillosis in a Gyr falcon. The highlighted heterophil contains intraplasmatic granules with central bodies.

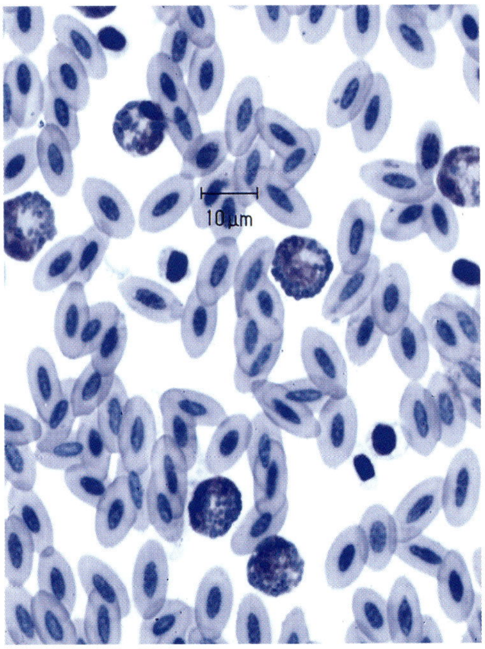

Figure 5.3: A Saker falcon with chronic aspergillosis. Six heterophils are visible which show different stages of altered granulation indicating toxic changes. Several thrombocytes are also present.

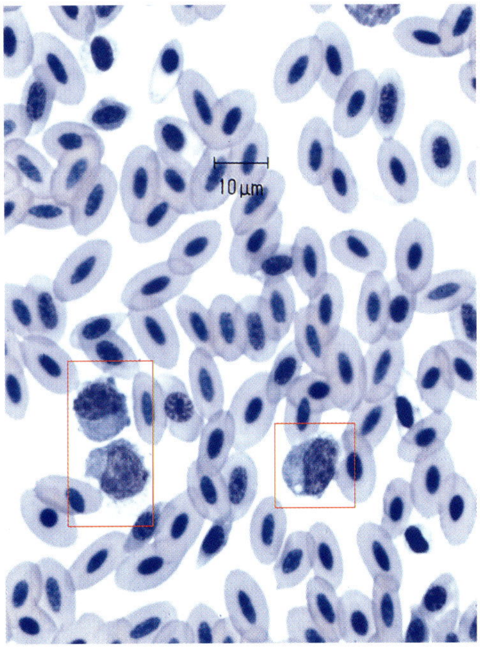

Figure 5.4: Three monocytes (highlighted) from a Gyr with subacute aspergillosis (WBC 14.0 x 10^9/l, 82 % heterophils, 2 % lymphocytes, 16 % monocytes).

5

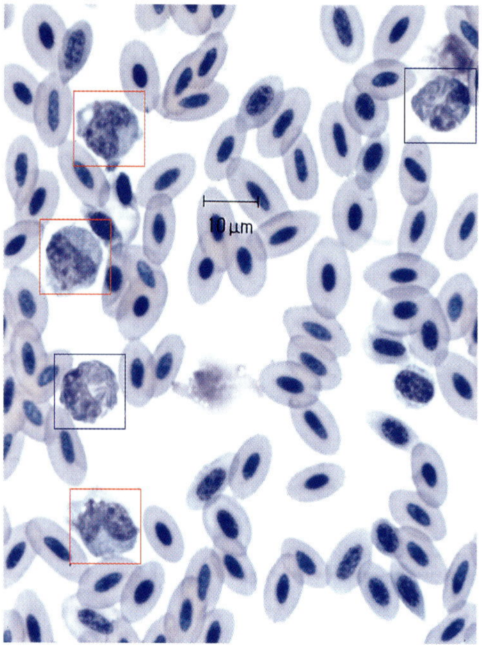

Figure 5.5: Two heterophils (highlighted in blue) and three reactive monocytes (highlighted in red) from a Gyr hybrid with chronic aspergillosis.

Aspergillosis

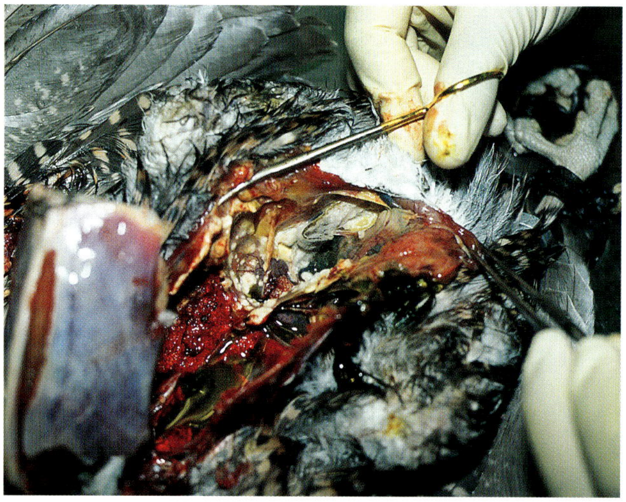

Figure 5.6: A Gyr falcon with generalized aspergillosis.

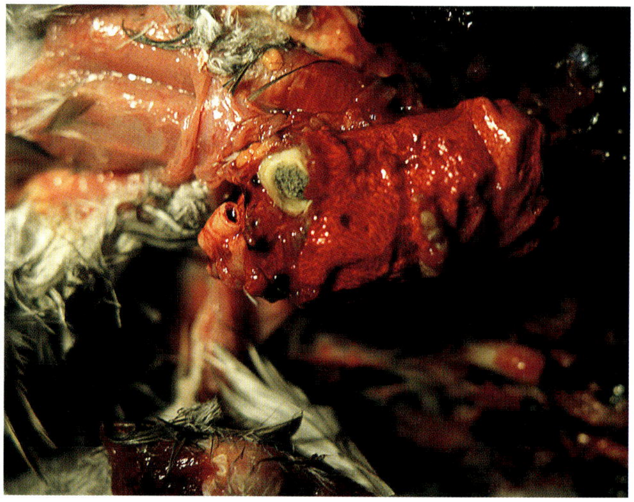

Figure 5.7: Fungal plaque on the lung of a Saker falcon.

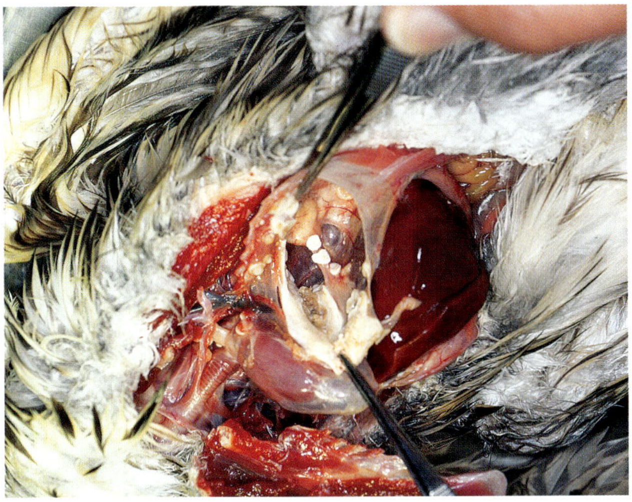

Figure 5.8: Grey to green fungal mats on the airsac wall of a Gyr falcon.

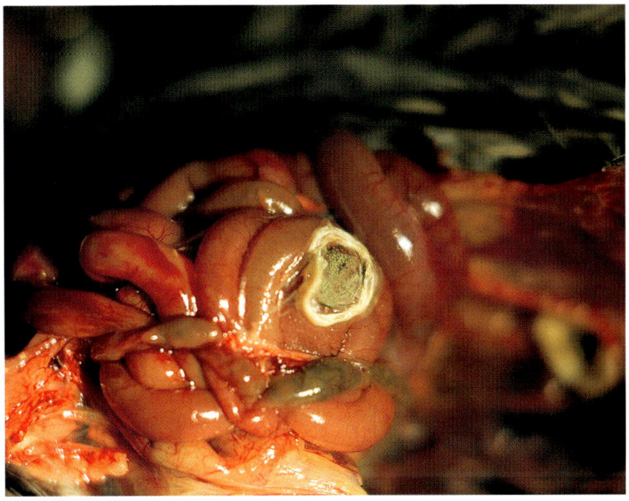

Figure 5.9: Fungal mat on the small intestine of a Gyr falcon.

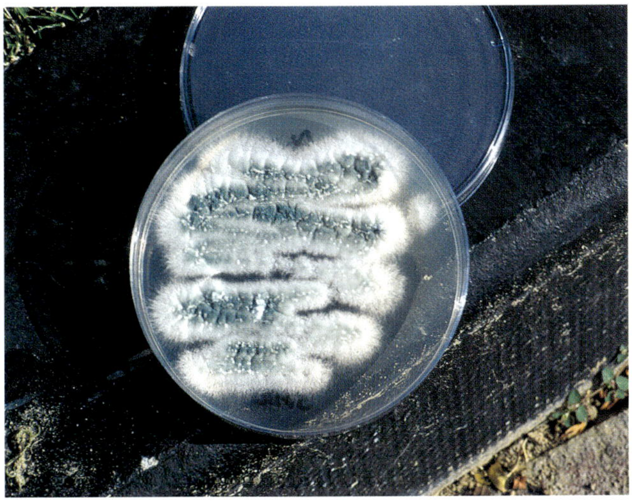

Figure 5.10 a: *A. fumigatus* on Sabourand agar.

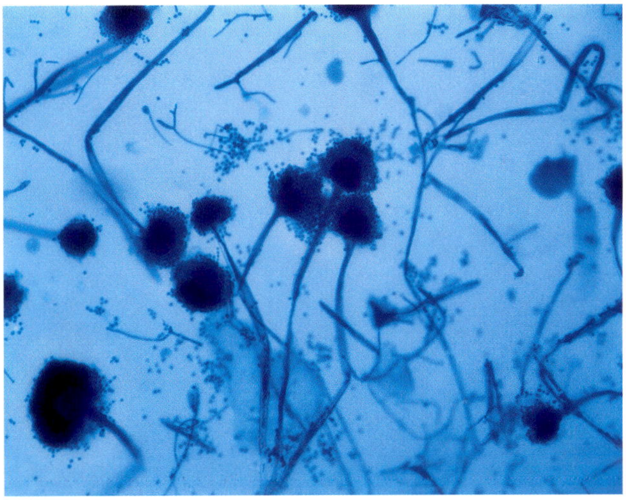

Figure 5.10 b: *A. fumigatus:* Methylene-blue stain from a colony.

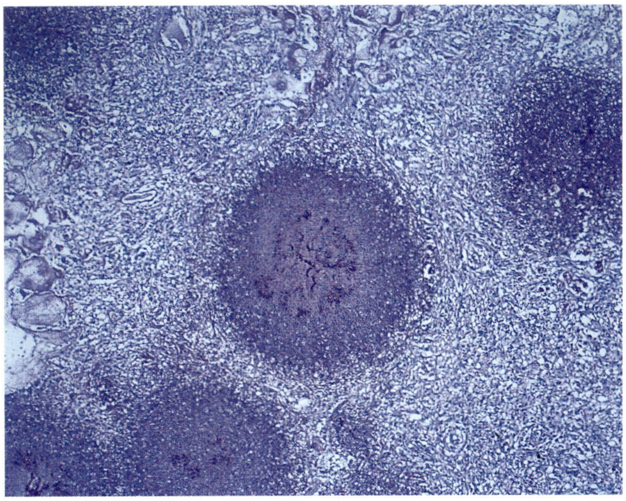

Figure 5.11: Pneumonia caused by *A. fumigatus* in a Peregrine falcon. Round eosinophilic foci containing numerous fungal hyphae. PAS stain.

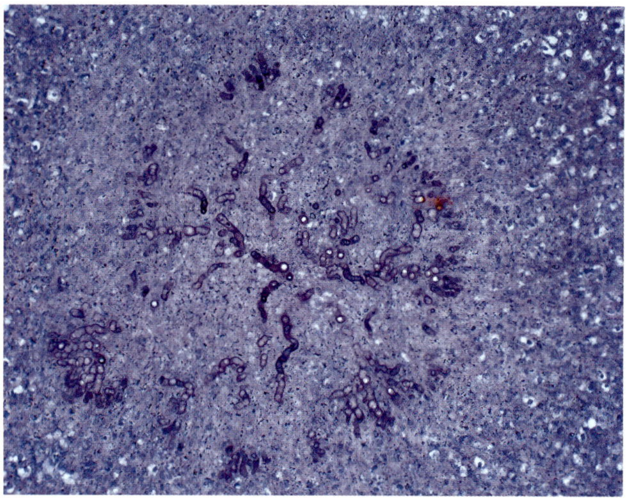

Figure 5.12: Granuloma of the same case as in Figure 5.11: Numerous dichotomously branched, septate fungal hyphae in the necrotic center of the granuloma branching to the periphery. PAS stain.

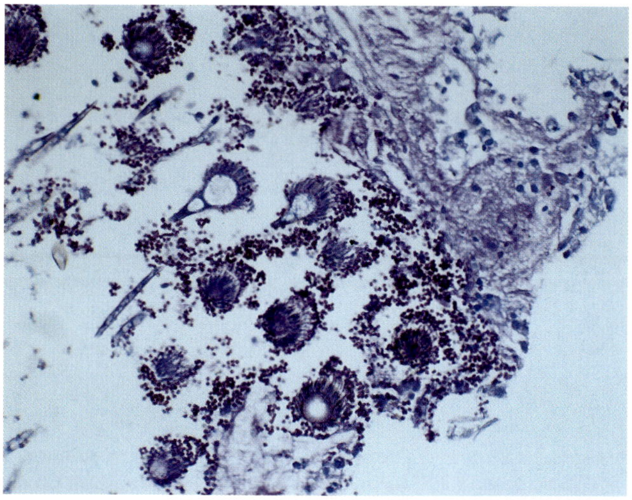

Figure 5.13: Conidiophores of *A. fumigatus* in the airsac space of a Gyr falcon. PAS stain.

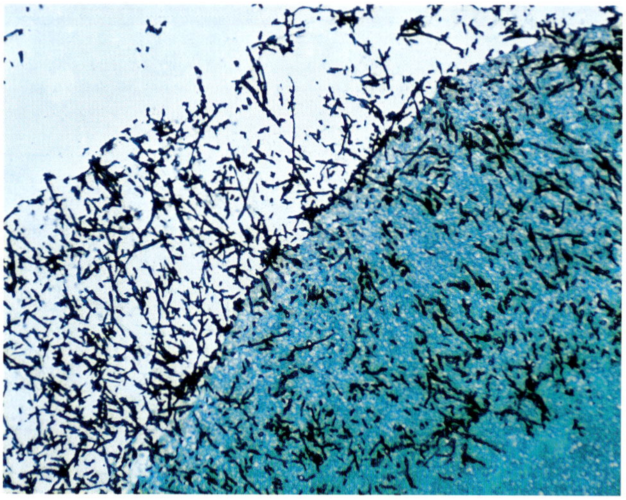

Figure 5.14: Numerous dark dichotomously branched fungal hyphae branching out of the necrotic airsac tissue of a Gyr hybrid. Grocott stain.

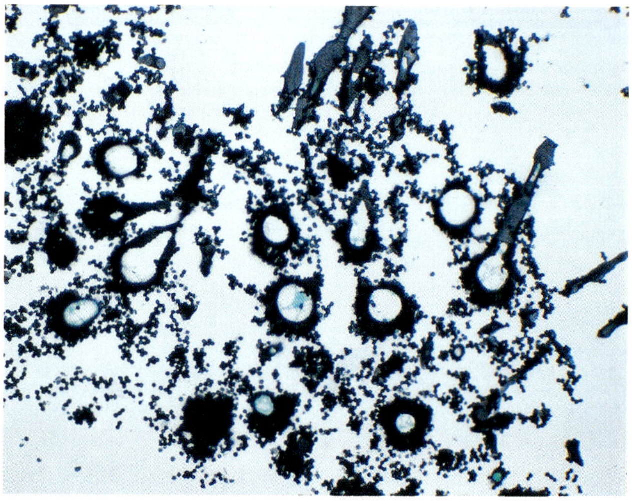

Figure 5.15: Conidiophores of *A. fumigatus* in the airsac space of a Gyr hybrid. Grocott stain.

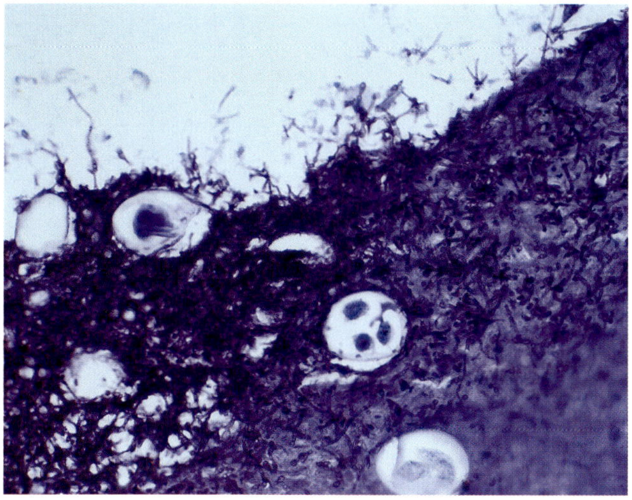

Figure 5.16: Airsac: Embryonated eggs of *Serratospiculum* spp. embedded between fungal hyphae of a Gyr falcon. *Serratospiculum* spp. infection may trigger aspergillosis. HE stain.

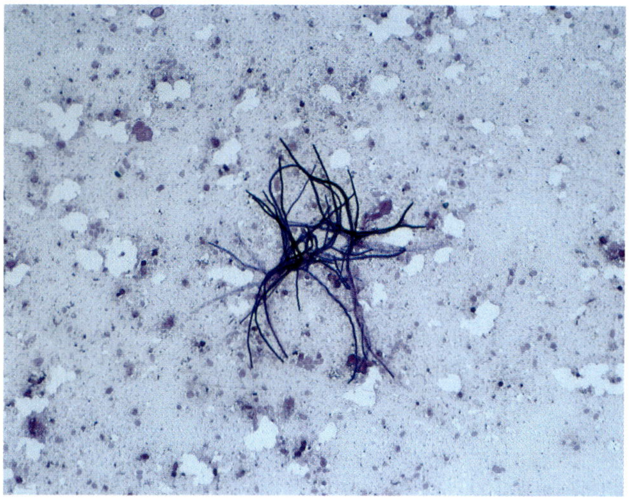

Figure 5.17: Airsac smear of a Peregrine falcon: typical fungal hyphae with some cellular debris. Gram stain.

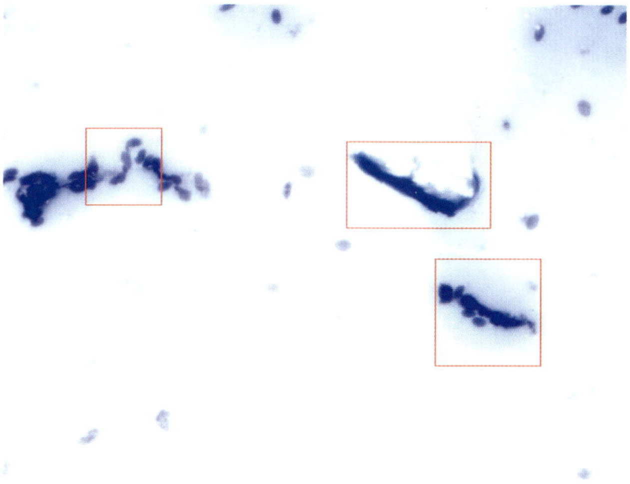

Figure 5.18: Airsac smear of a Gyr falcon: Fibrin strands (highlighted), few epithelial cells and erythrocytes. It may sometimes be difficult to distinguish between fungal hyphae and fibrin strands. Gram stain.

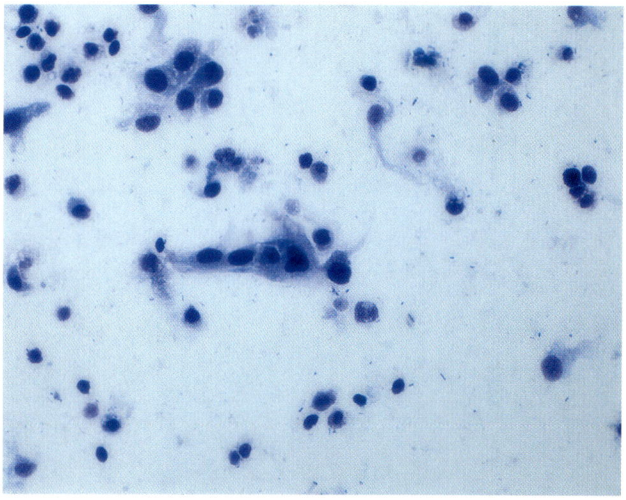

Figure 5.19: Bacterial airsacculitis of a Saker falcon. No hyphae are visible, however many Gram-positive rods can be seen. Gram stain.

5

Other fungal diseases

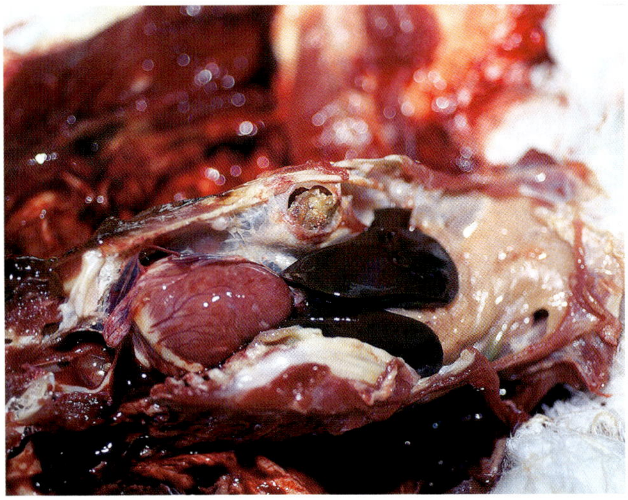

Figure 5.20: White Gyr falcon with a large granuloma in the left caudal airsac, caused by *A. nidulans*

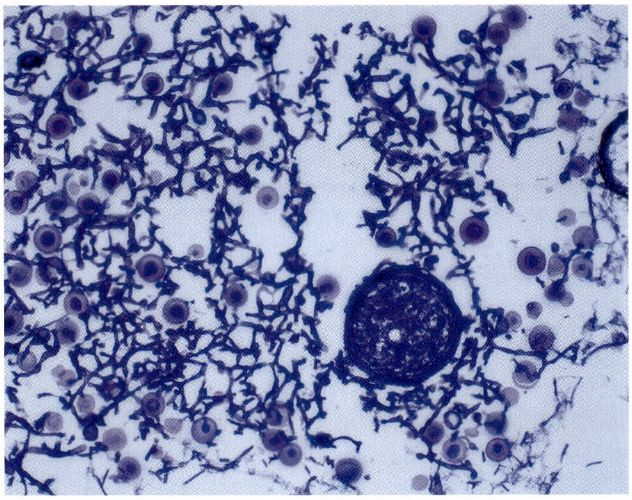

Figure 5.21: Airsac of a white Gyr falcon: Necrotic material and numerous fungal hyphae with conidiophores. PAS stain.

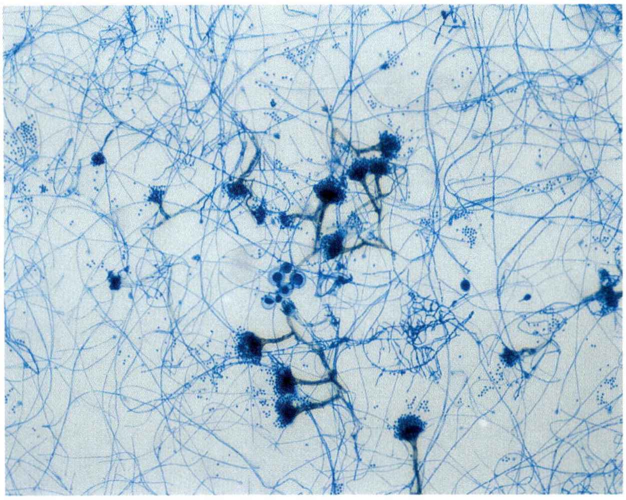

Figure 5.22: *Emericella nidulans*, the teleomorph of *A. nidulans* in the airsac of a white Gyr falcon. PAS stain.

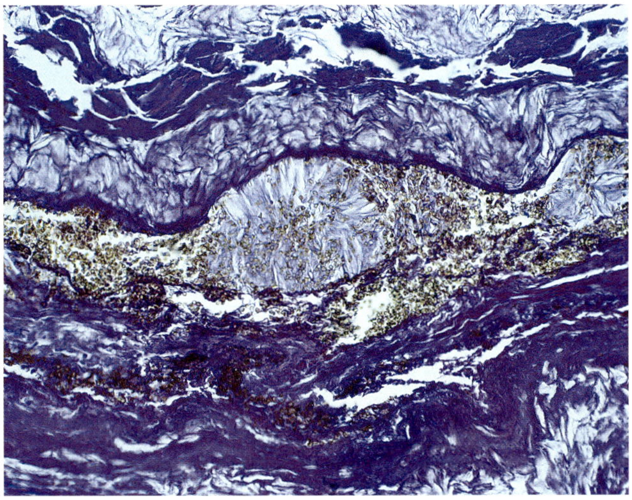

Figure 5.23: Airsac mycosis: Female Gyr falcon with numerous round brownish organisms in the airsac space. PAS stain.

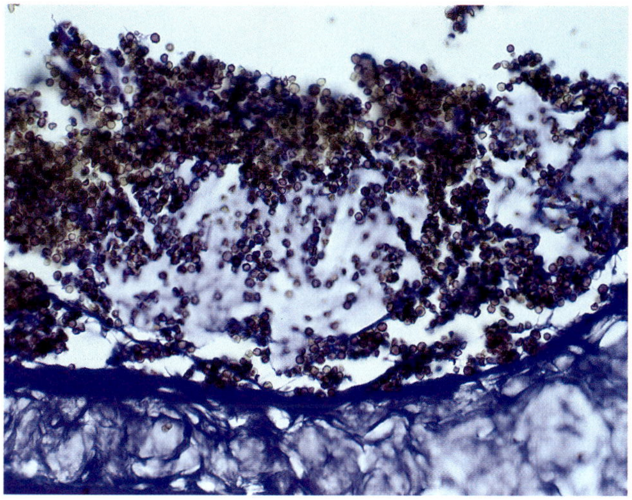

Figure 5.24: Airsac mycosis: Higher magnification of Figure 5.23 with numerous round yeast-like cells suspected to be *Blastomyces* spp. No hyphae visible. PAS stain.

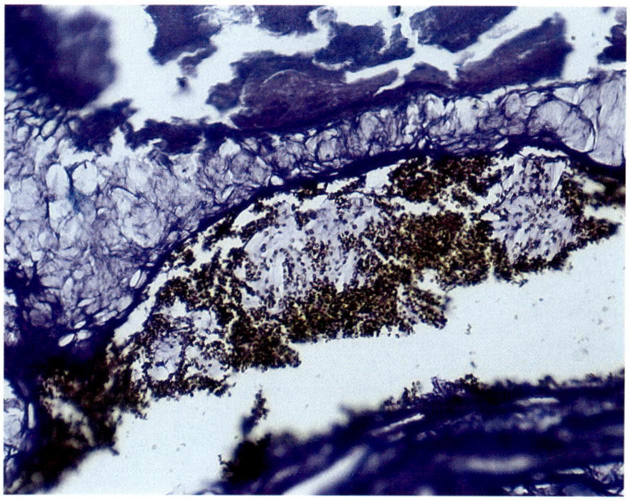

Figure 5.25: Oesophageal zygomycosis: Crop of a female Saker falcon with diphtheroid inflammation and numerous irregular, non-septate, randomly branched hyphae. This type of fungal hyphae is consistent with a zygomycete infection. PAS stain.

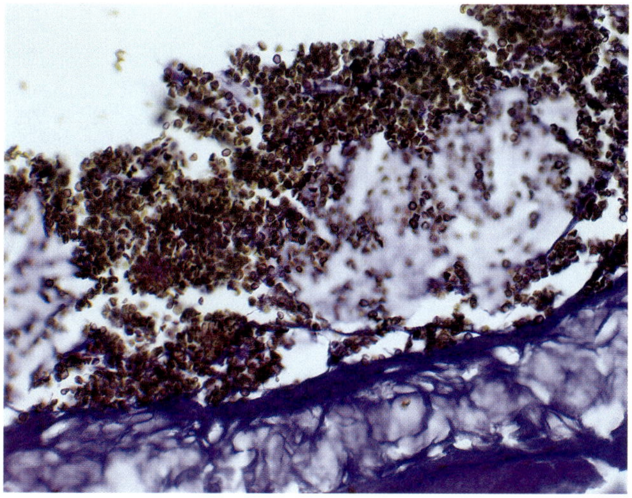

Figure 5.26: Oesophageal zygomycosis: Same case as shown in Figure 5.25. With a HE-stained preparation, hyphae are more difficult to detect, but appear as rounded features with a distinct border. However, special stains are required to confirm mycosis.

5

Candidiasis

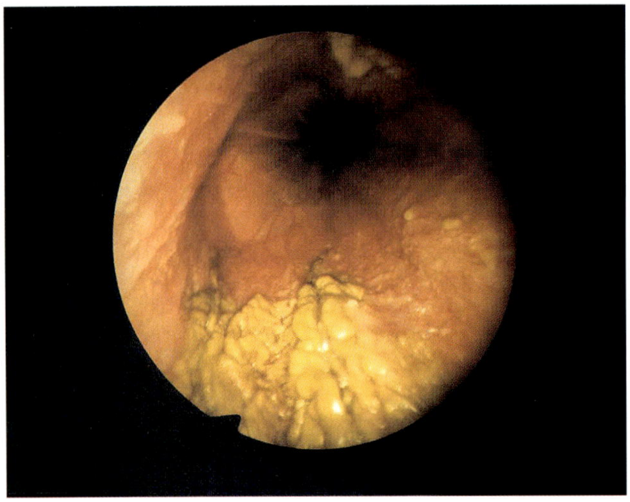

Figure 5.27 a: Endoscopic view of the crop of a Saker falcon (*Falco cherrug*) affected with clinical candidiasis. Note the yellowish colour of the mucous membrane. Atypical clinical signs included reduced appetite, regurgitation and weight loss.

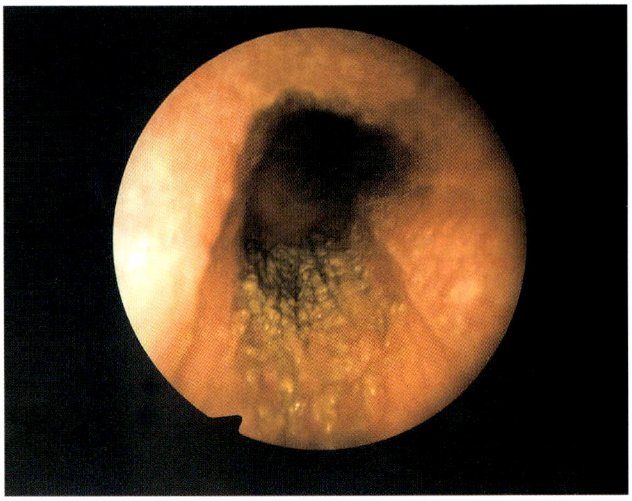

Figure 5.27 b: Another endoscopic view of the crop of the same Saker falcon (*Falco cherrug*) as in the previous figure.

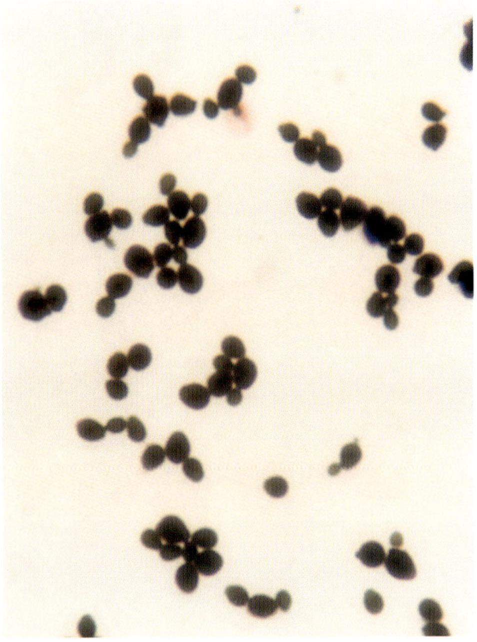

Figure 5.28 a: Gram stained smear of *Candida albicans* budding yeast cells.

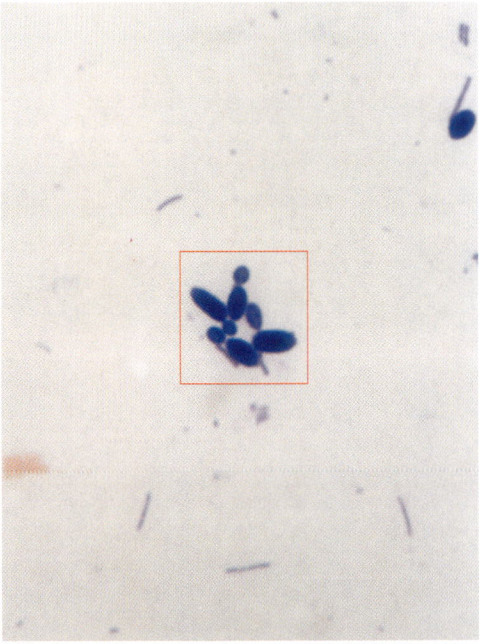

Figure 5.28 b: Direct smear from the crop of a Saker falcon (*Falco cherrug*), infected with candidiasis. Wet swabs are taken from the crop and stained with Rapid Romanowsky stain. Budding yeast cells are seen in the smear (highlighted) and long bacterial rods.

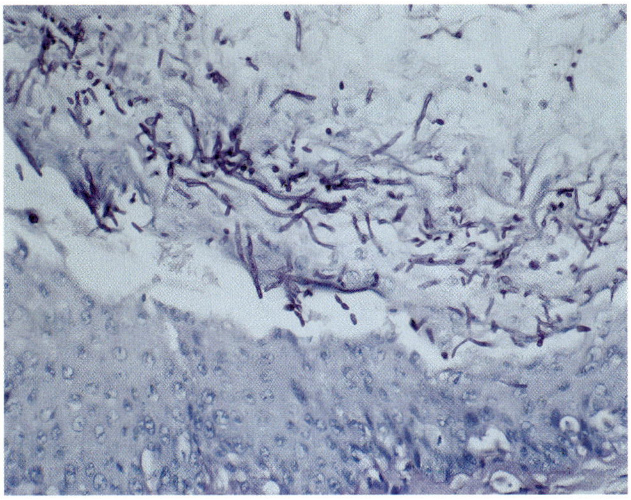

Figure 5.29: Oesophagitis caused by *Candida albicans:* Crop of a Gyr falcon with cellular debris containing numerous pseudohyphae and blastospores attached to the mucosa. PAS stain.

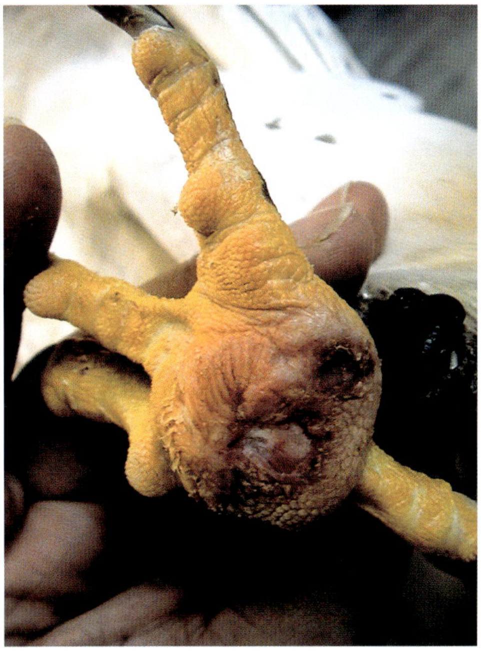

Figure 5.30: Nine-year-old Gyr falcon with severe chronic bumblefoot causing marked swelling of the plantar surface of the foot. In addition to alimentary tract infections *Candida albicans* is often involved in pododermatitis (bumblefoot) and other skin infections.

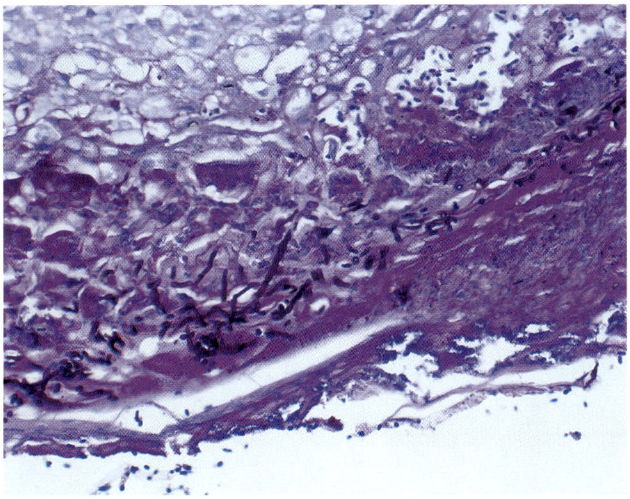

Figure 5.31: Pododermatitis of a Saker falcon: Chronic pyogranulative dermatitis caused by *Candida albicans*, demonstrating numerous pseudohyphae and blastospores in the debris. PAS stain.

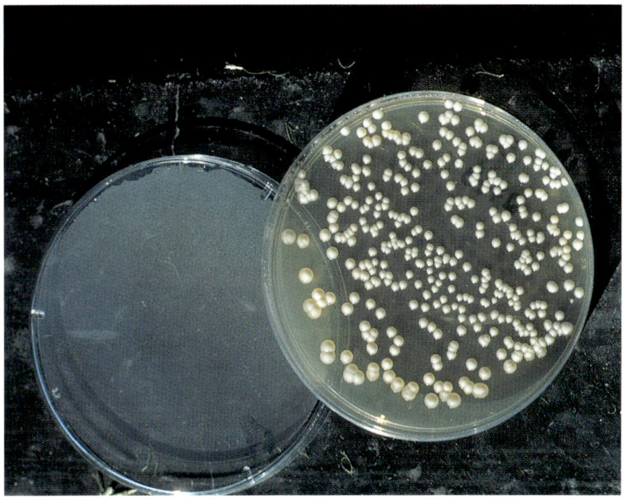

Figure 5.32: Growth of *Candida albicans* on Sabouraud agar.

Chapter 6

Parasitic Diseases

Protozoa

Protozoal diseases are common in falcons and only the most important ones are presented here. Because haematology and biochemistry values are, with few exceptions, not significantly altered from reference values, no values are shown. One exception is malaria, where often haemolytic anaemias are observed. It is worthwhile mentioning that a circulating eosinophilia is rare in relation to parasitic diseases in falcons.

Haemoprotozoa

Malaria

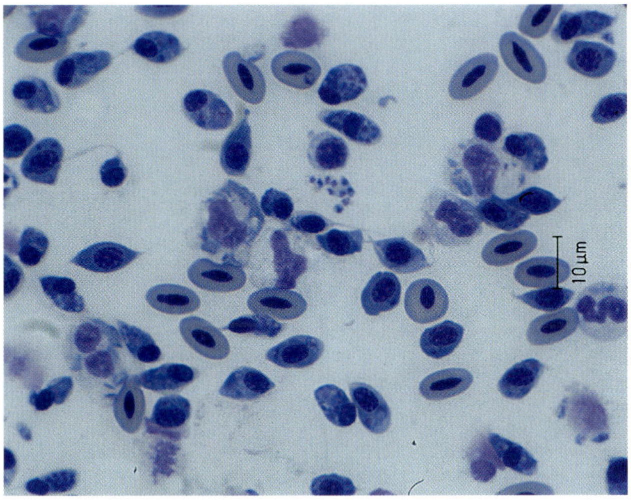

Figure 6.1: Peregrine falcon with severe haemolytic anaemia showing polychromasia, anisocytosis, poikilocytosis and hyperchromasia. Parasites of the genus *Plasmodium* cause avian malaria and mosquitoes (*Culex*, *Aedes*) serve as intermediate hosts.

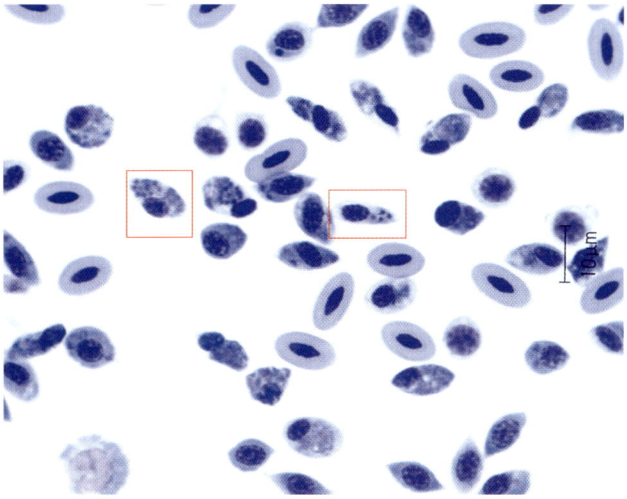

Figure 6.2: A preparation of the same falcon as shown in Figure 6.1. *Plasmodium relictum* schizonts and gametocytes are seen in the cytoplasm of erythrocytes. The organism can also be found in thrombocytes and leukocytes. This Gyr hybrid falcon showed the following blood picture: RBC 1.8 x 10^{12} /l, HB 7.8 g/dl, WBC 10.2 x 10^{9}/l.

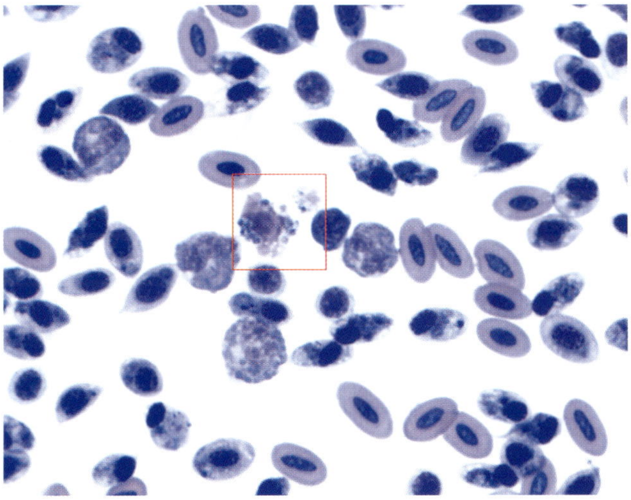

Figure 6.3: *Plasmodium relictum* (like Figures 6.1 and 6.2) has a world-wide distribution in many avian families and in some it is pathogenic and often fatal. Many erythrocytes contain the parasite, some of which have burst and released the gametocytes.

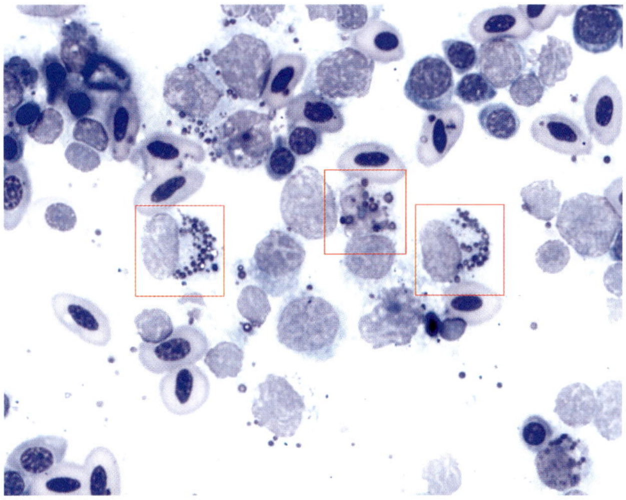

Figure 6.4: Three heterophils with severe destruction caused by *P. relictum* infection of the same Gyr hybrid falcon.

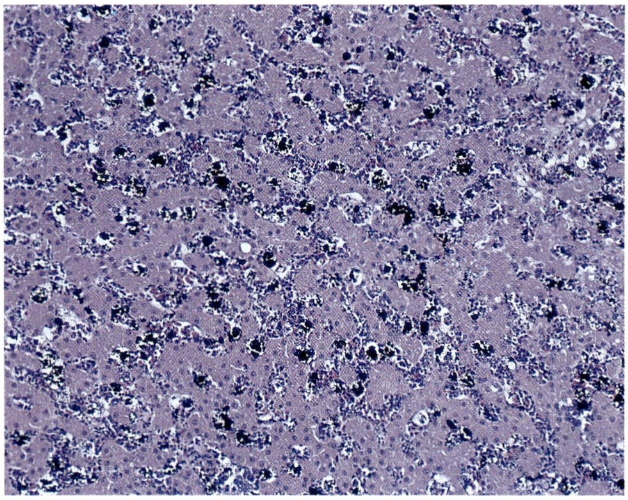

Figure 6.5: Deposit of haematin malaria pigment in Kupffer cells in the liver of the same Gyr hybrid. This is the only pathognomonic lesion in cases of malaria. As described for other avians, schizonts in Kupffer cells and mononuclear hepatitis are rarely observed in falcons. HE stain.

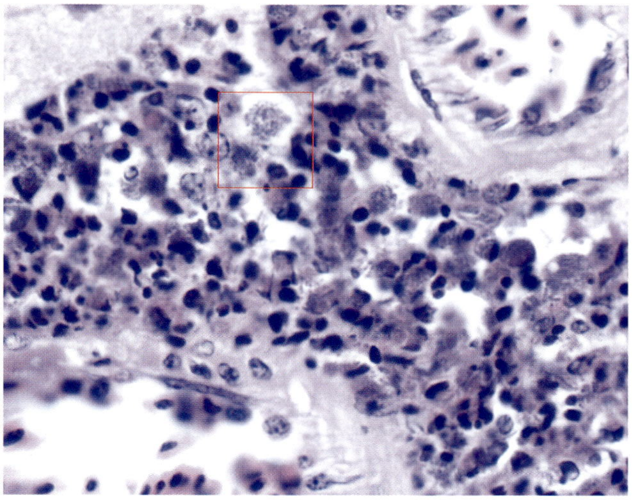

Figure 6.6: Nonsuppurative perivascular focal encephalitis with schizont-like organisms most probably inside macrophages of a Gyr falcon. This finding is suggestive of malaria. HE stain.

Babesiosis

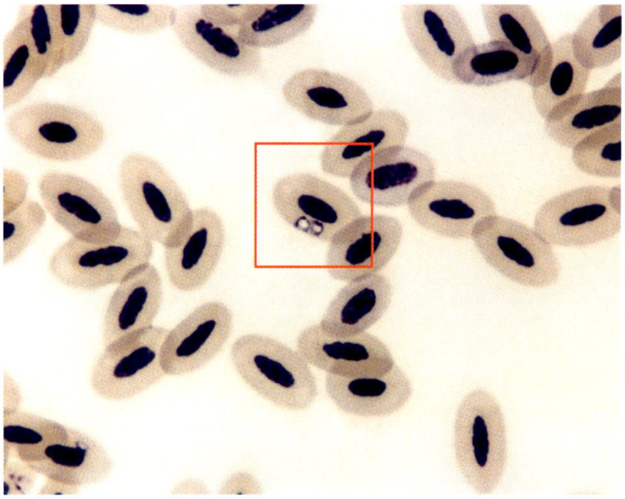

Figure 6.7: *Babesia shortti* in the cytoplasm of an erythrocyte from a Saker falcon (*Falco cherrug*), (modified Wright Giemsa stain).

Haemoproteosis

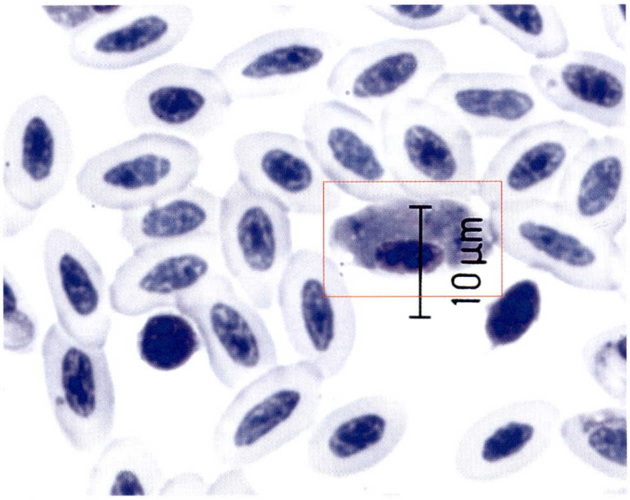

Figure 6.8: *Haemoproteus* spp. in the cytoplasm of erythrocytes of a Gyr falcon. These are erythrocytic gametocytes which practically encircle the erythrocyte nucleus (»halter-shaped« appearance).

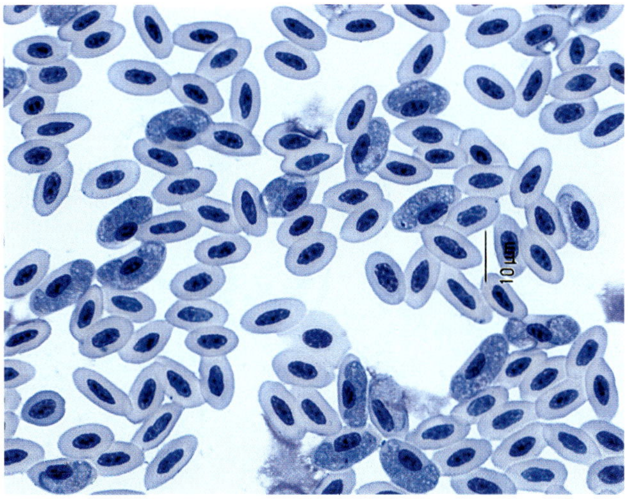

Figure 6.9: Heavy infection with *Haemoproteus* spp. in a Peregrine falcon. The parasite is transmitted by blood-sucking insects like hippoboscid fly. The number of gametocytes seen in peripheral blood varies with stress, season and age.

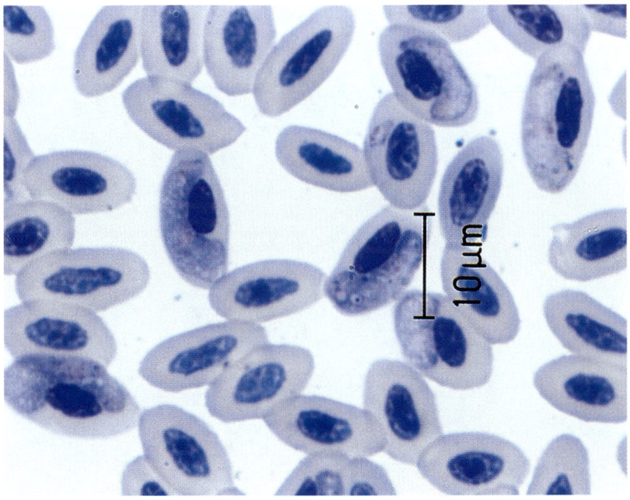

Figure 6.10: *Haemoproteus tinnunculi* infection (courteously identified by Dr. O. Krone, IZW, Berlin, Germany) in a Saker falcon. This parasite is minimally, if at all pathogenic in falcons.

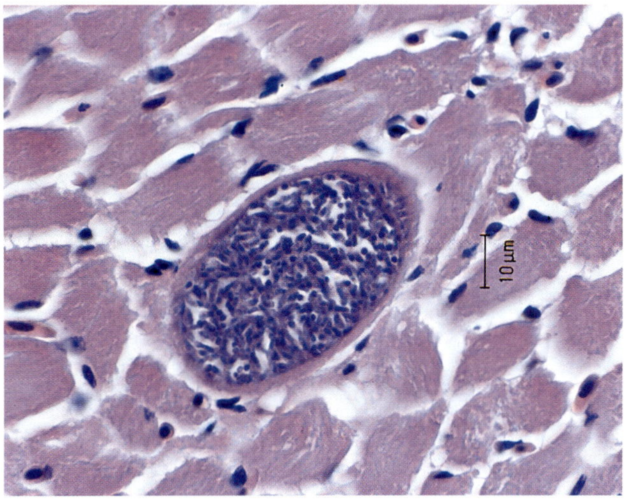

Figure 6.11: Haemoproteosis of the muscle: Large parasitic cyst (megaloschizont of *Haemoproteus* spp., courteously identified by Dr. O. Krone, IZW, Berlin, Germany) located between muscle fibres. No inflammation is present. The differentiation of these cysts from *Sarcocystis* or *Leucocytozoon* cysts is difficult. HE stain.

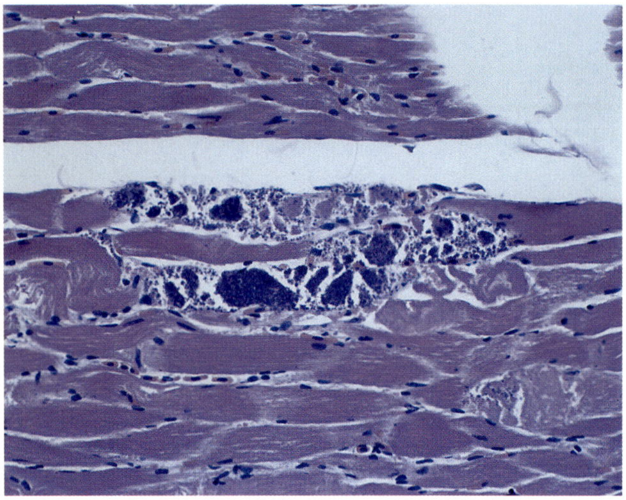

Figure 6.12: Haemoproteosis of muscle: Calcified parasitic cyst with focal reactive myositis. The calcified structures are most probably residues of the parasite. Their pathogenicity is unknown, however in cases with myositis poor performance may occur. HE stain.

6

Leucocytozoonosis

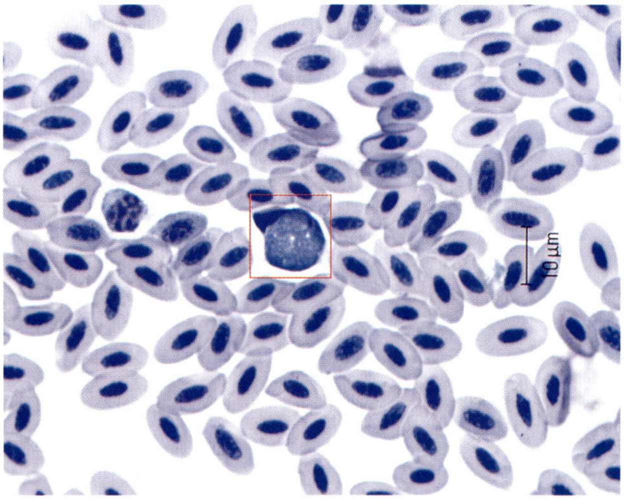

Figure 6.13: A *Leucocytozoon* parasite in a Gyr falcon. This is a gametocyte.

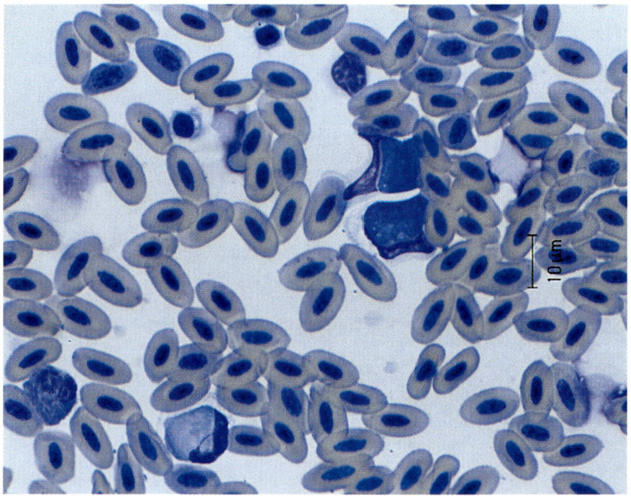

Figure 6.14: Two *Leucocytozoon* macro gametocytes in the blood of a Saker falcon. This parasite is minimally, if at all pathogenic in falcons and is transmitted by black flies (Simulidae).

Protozoa of the alimentary tract

Trichomonosis (Frounce)

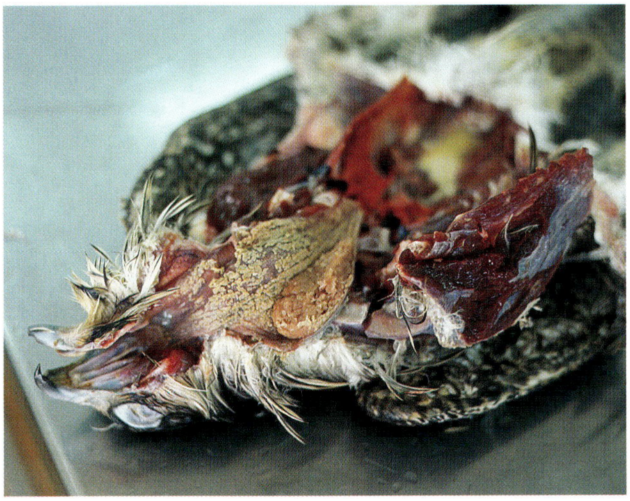

Figure 6.15: A Saker falcon with typical lesions of Trichomonosis in the pharynx and crop.

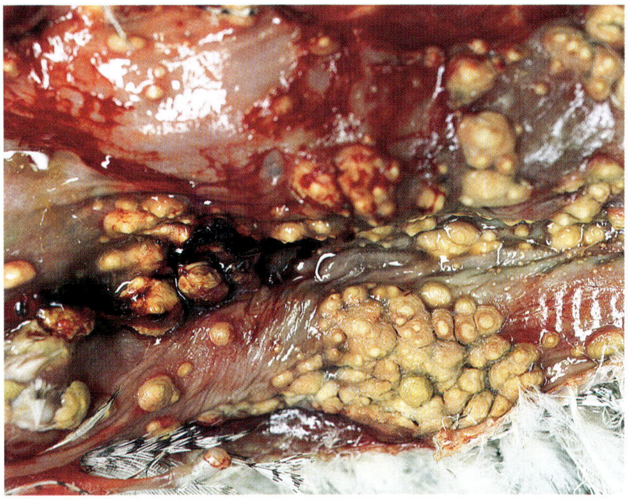

Figure 6.16: *Trichomonas gallinae* nodules in the pharynx and crop of a Gyr hybrid. Falcons contract trichomonosis or frounce by ingesting infected pigeons.

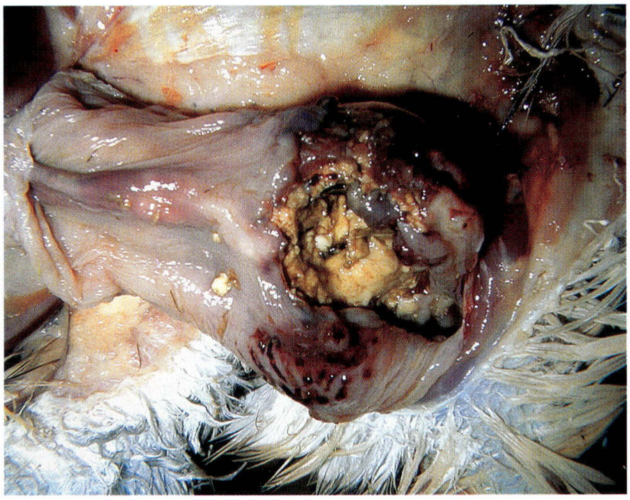

Figure 6.17: Necrotizing lesion in the crop of a Peregrine x Gyr hybrid. Such severe lesions are rare in falcons.

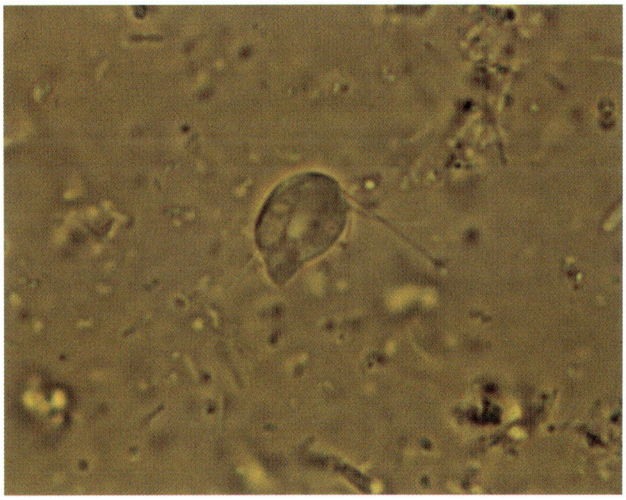

Figure 6.18: *Trichomonas gallinae* from the pharynx of a Saker falcon.

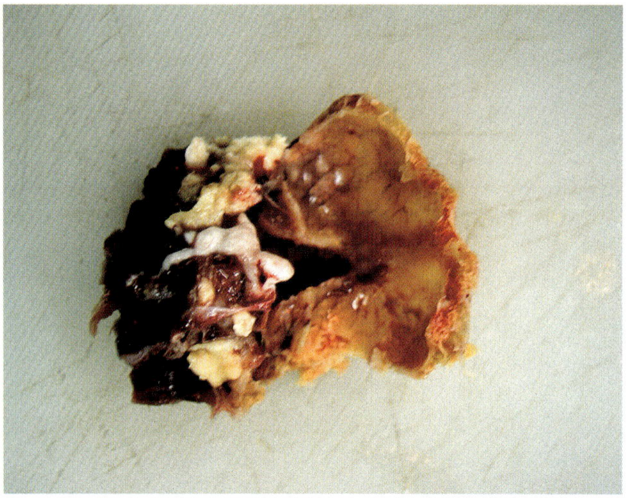

Figure 6.19: Caseous mass observed in both ear canals of a Saker falcon. This lesion is suggestive of trichomonosis.

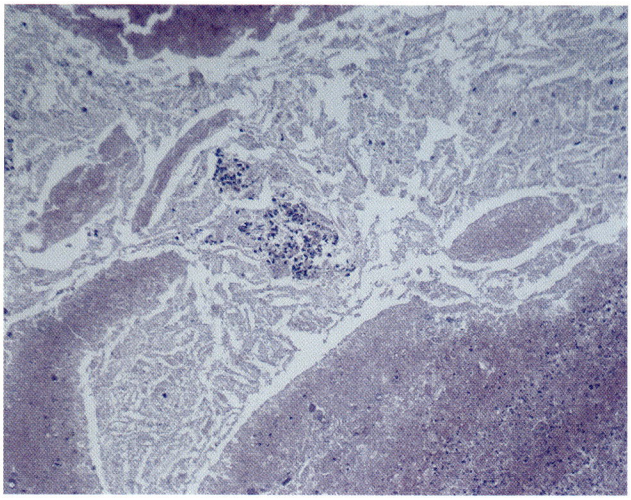

Figure 6.20: Otitis: Massive necrosis most probably caused by *Trichomonas gallinae*. However, it is difficult to find the parasites due to their rapid disintegration following death. HE stain.

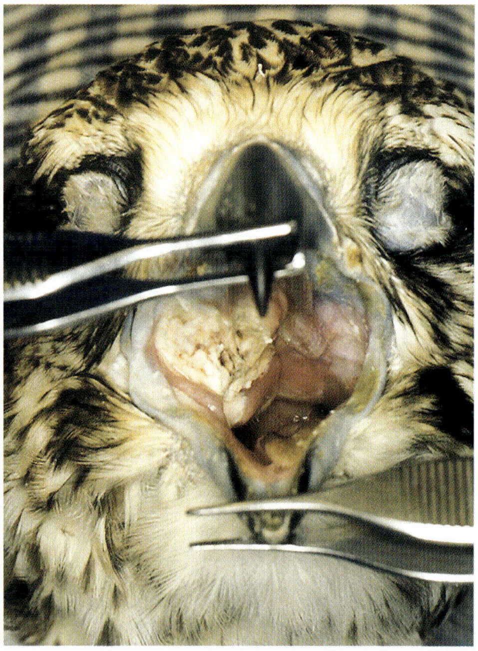

Figure 6.21: Large trichomonosis growth on the dorsolateral aspect of the oropharynx of a Saker falcon (*Falco cherrug*).

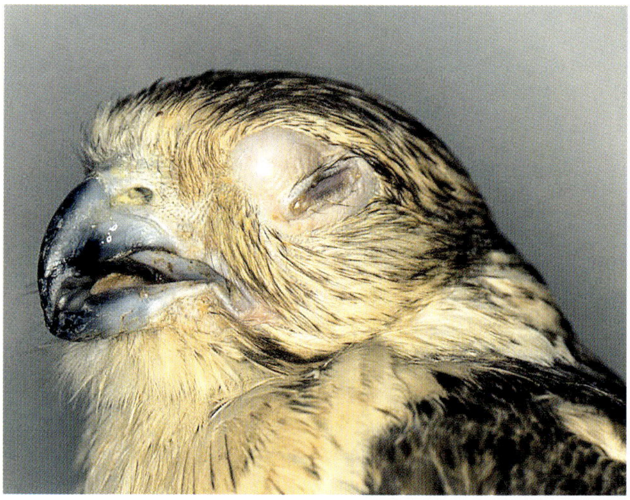

Figure 6.22: *Trichomonas* infection affecting the supraorbital diverticulum of the infraorbital sinus in a Saker falcon (*Falco cherrug*).

Flagellate enteritis

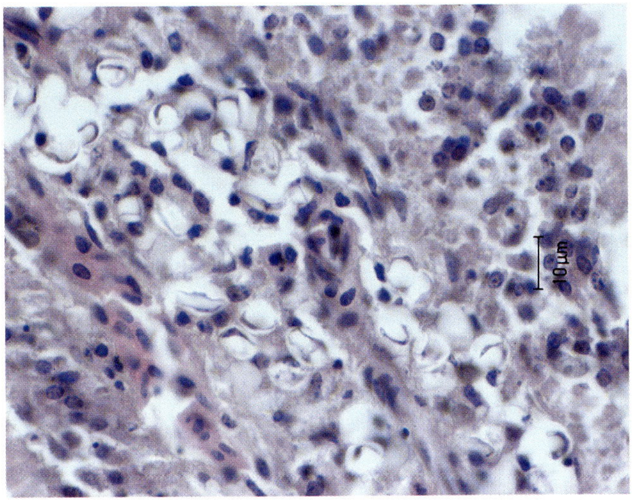

Figure 6.23: Protozoal enteritis: Flagellate infection is very rare in falcons and in this case no clinical signs were observed. Lymphoplasmocytic infiltration of the mucosa is caused by numerous comma-shaped organisms (species not identified) in a small intestinal crypt. The organism is difficult to see in HE-stained sections. HE stain.

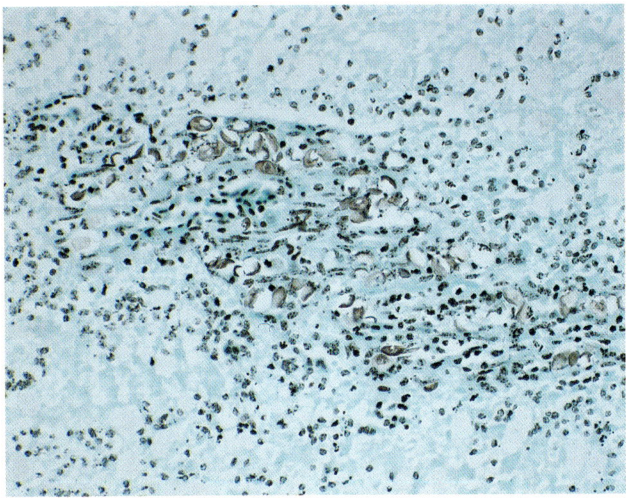

Figure 6.24: Protozoal enteritis: In silver-stained sections, shape and size of the flagellate-organisms are clearly visible due to the argyrophylic reaction of the protozoa. Grocott stain.

6

Coccidiosis

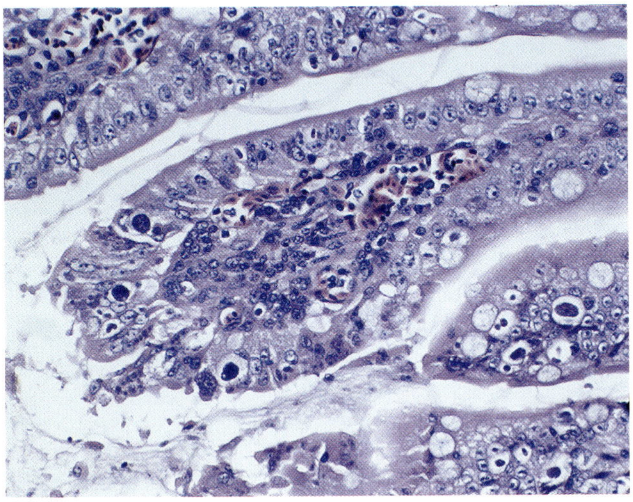

Figure 6.25: Catarrhal enteritis of a Barbary falcon (*Falco pelegrinoides*) caused by chronic *Caryospora* sp. infection. *Caryospora* sp. coccidiosis is a problem in young and captive falcons, while adult birds develop some degree of immunity. Affected birds are usually stressed as a result of training or hunting and may develop diarrhoea. HE stain.

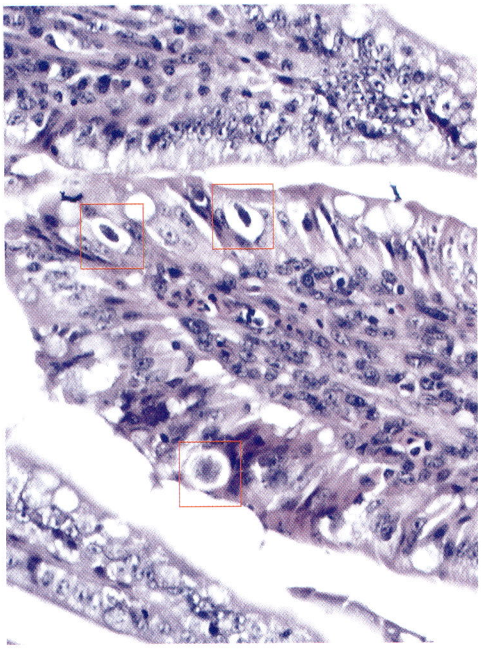

Figure 6.26: Coccidial enteritis: Numerous coccidian-stages (gamonts, oocysts) in the mucosa of the small intestine of a Gyr x Peregrine hybrid. HE stain.

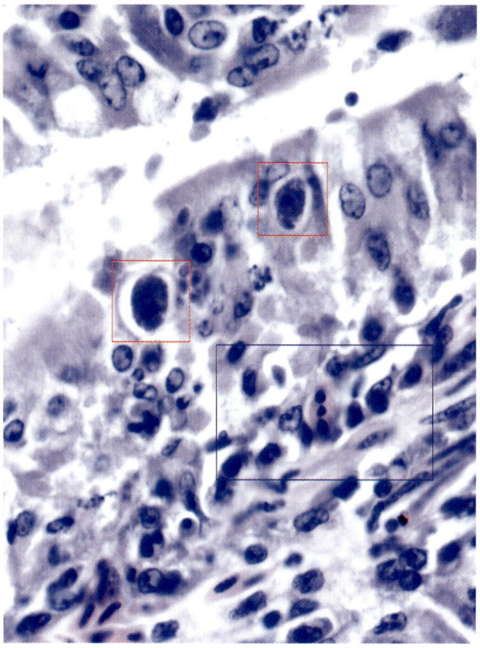

Figure 6.27: Coccidial enteritis in a Gyr falcon: Lymphoplasmocytic infiltration (highlighted in blue) of the *Lamina propria* beneath macrogamonts (highlighted in red). HE stain.

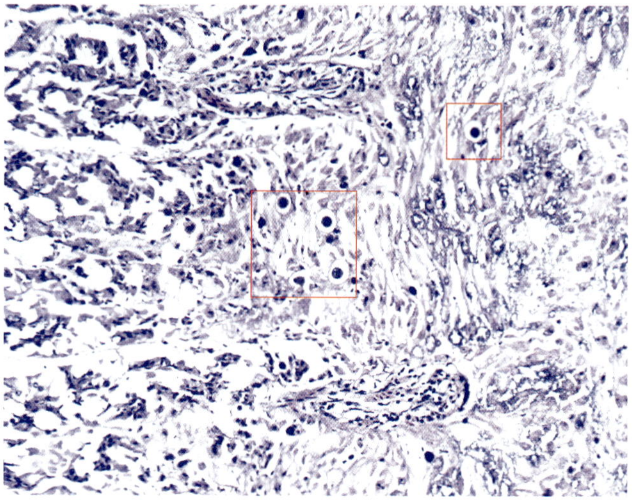

Figure 6.28: Coccidial enteritis and clostridiosis: Numerous oocysts (highlighted) in the intestinal lumen of a Peregrine falcon. Degenerated and necrotic intestinal mucosa is caused by synergistic clostridiosis. HE stain.

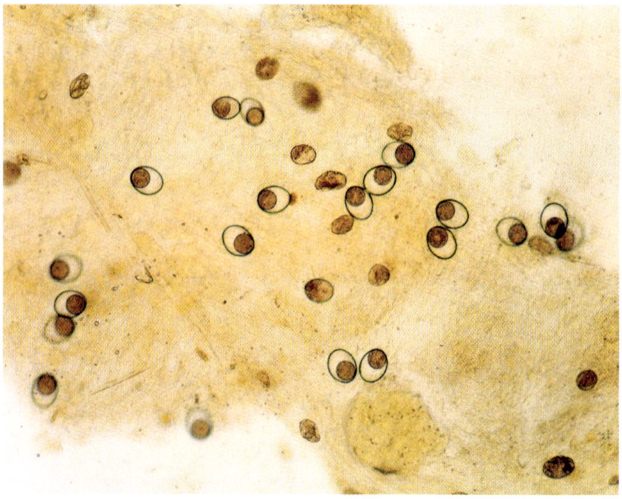

Figure 6.29 a: *Caryospora kutzeri* in faeces: Large number of unsporulated oocysts at 10 x from a Saker falcon (*Falco cherrug*).

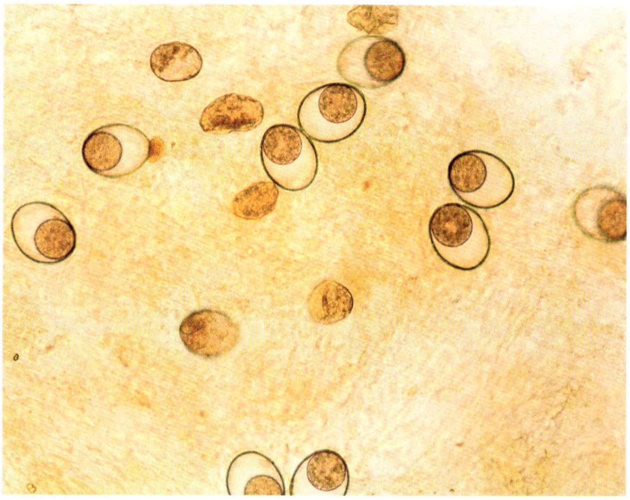

Figure 6.29 b: *Caryospora kutzeri* in faeces: Large number of unsporulated oocysts at 20 x from a Saker falcon.

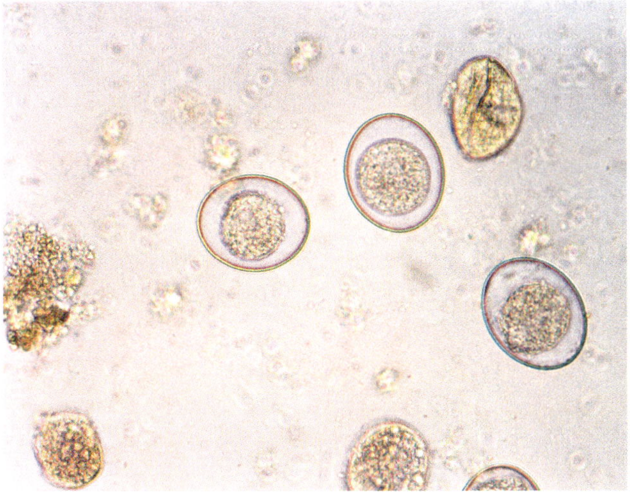

Figure 6.29 c: *Caryospora kutzeri* in faeces: Three unsporulated oocysts from a Saker falcon.

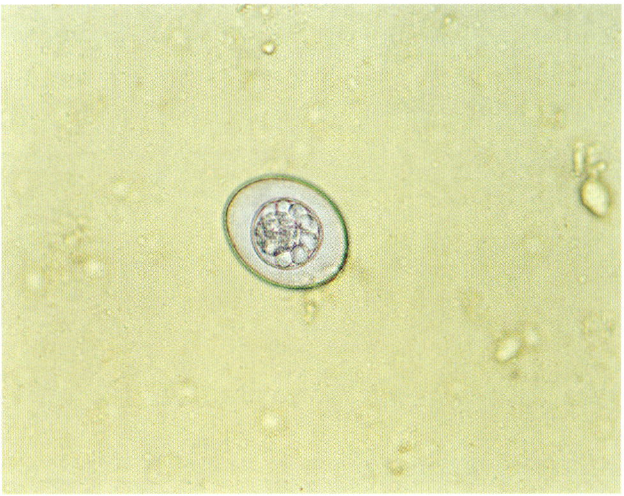

Figure 6.29 d: *Caryospora kutzeri* in faeces: One sporulated oocyst from a Saker falcon

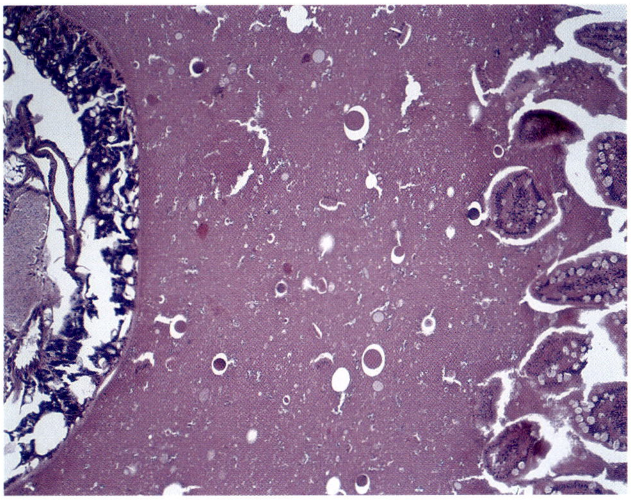

Figure 6.30: Coccidial enteritis and helminthosis: Numerous coccidian stages in the intestinal lumen of a Gyr falcon adjacent to a large unidentified round worm. HE stain.

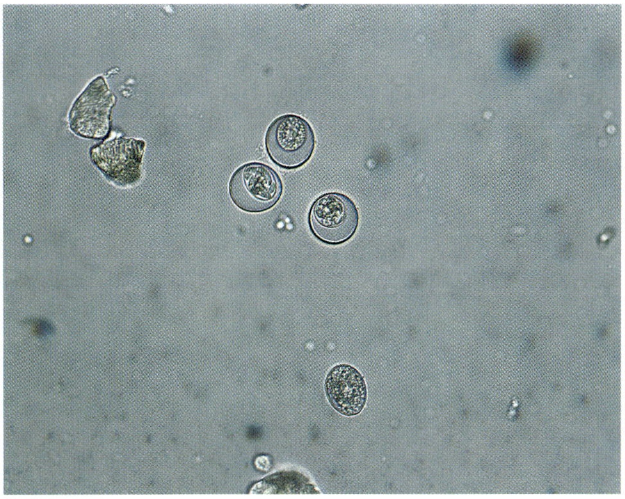

Figure 6.31: *Caryospora falconis* in faeces: Unsporulated oocysts of oval shape, containing a central granulated mass (sporont), 25 x 30 µm in size. Sporulated *Caryospora* sp. oocysts containing 1 sporocyst with 8 sporozoites. HE stain.

Helminths

Serratospiculosis

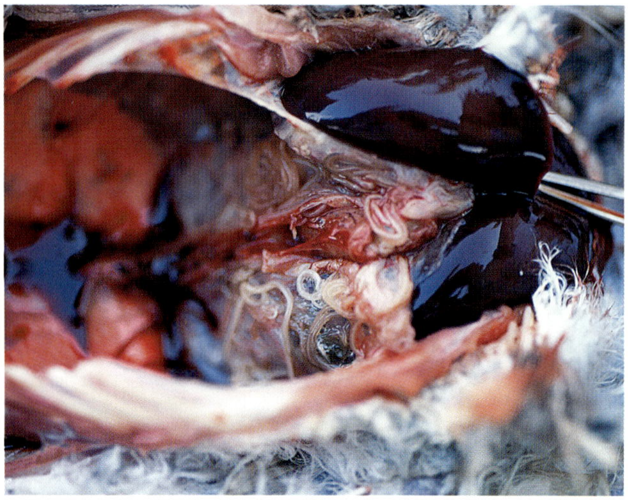

Figure 6.32: An aggregation of *Serratospiculum* sp. parasites in the airsac of a necropsied Peregrine falcon. In many necropsied falcons, or in falcons endoscoped for detection of aspergillosis, lesions caused by *Serratospiculum* sp. parasites are often detected. HE stain.

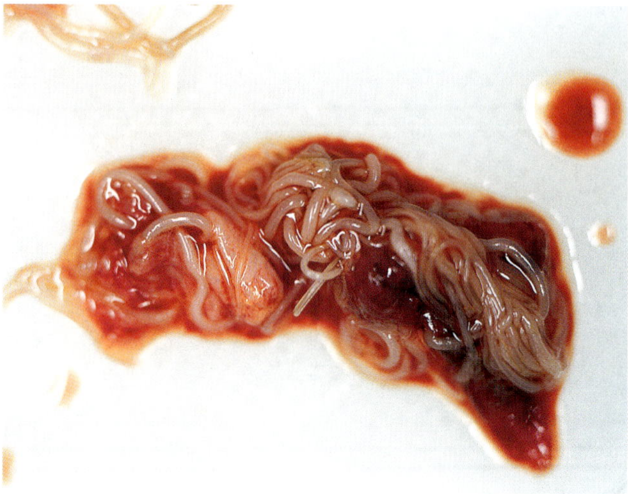

Figure 6.33: Numerous *Serratospiculum* sp. parasites from the airsac of a Gyr falcon. In the Middle East, *S. seurati* is the most common falcon parasite. HE stain.

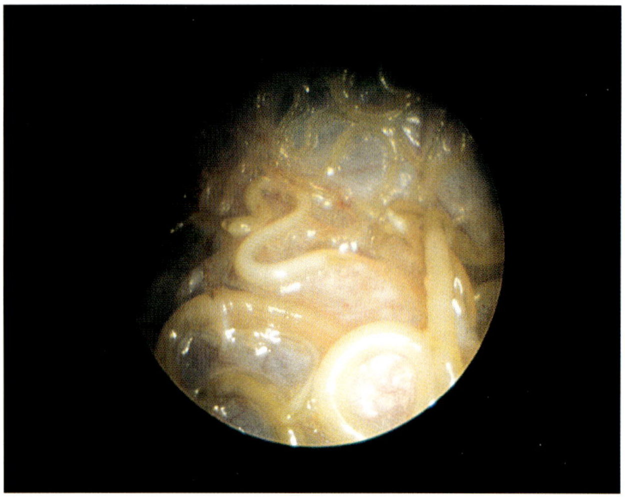

Figure 6.34: Large numbers of adult *Serratospiculum* sp. filarial nematodes in the abdominal airsac of a falcon observed during endoscopic examination. The abdominal air sacs seem to be the preferred site of adult *Serratospiculum* sp. parasitic colonisation.

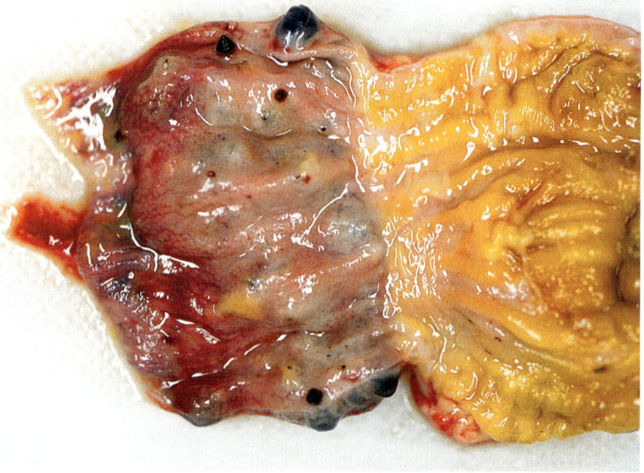

Figure 6.35: Proventriculus of a Gyr falcon with some haemorrhagic nodules. After ingestion of infected insects, the *Serratospiculum* L3 larva penetrates the wall of the proventriculus and develops into the adult filarial parasite within the airsac.

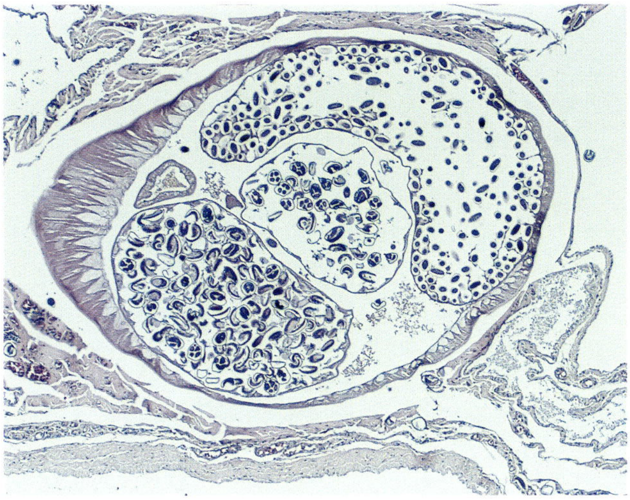

Figure 6.36: Adult *Serratospiculum* sp. parasite attached to the airsac wall. The uterus of the parasite contains numerous embryonated eggs. HE stain.

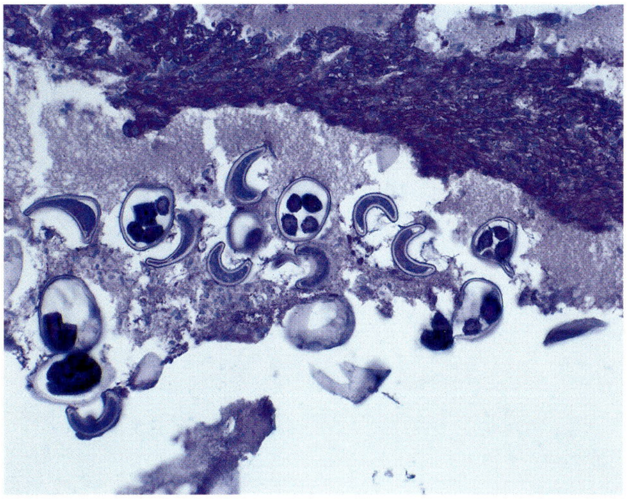

Figure 6.37: Numerous embryonated *Serratospiculum* sp. eggs surrounded by fibrinous material attached to the air sac wall. PAS stain.

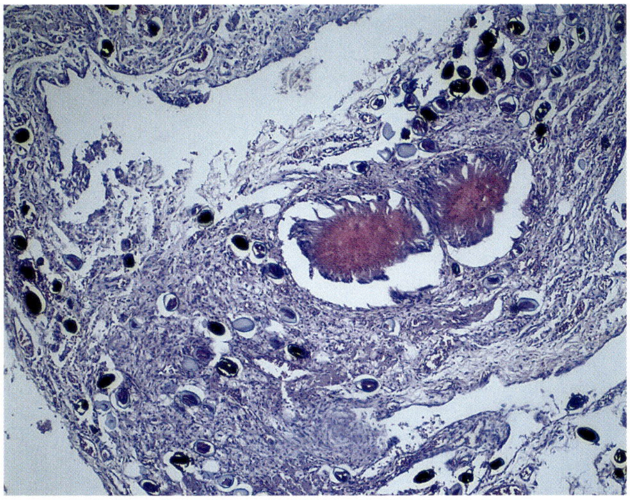

Figure 6.38: Air sac necrosis surrounded by fibrinous exudates containing numerous embryonated *Serratospiculum* sp. eggs. The pathogencity of the parasite is unclear, however an associated significant inflammatory reaction may reduce performance. PAS stain.

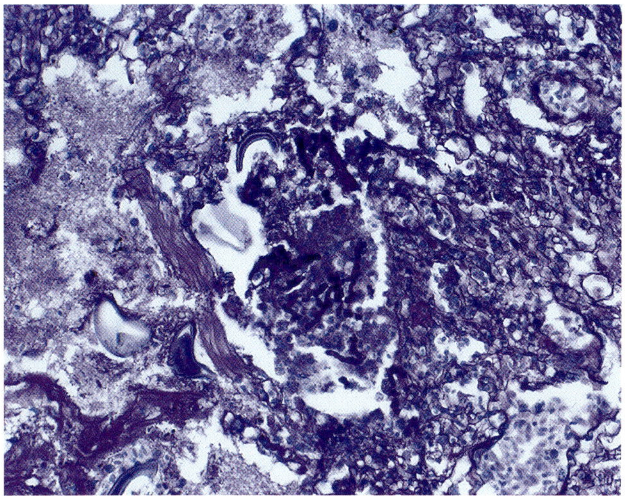

Figure 6.39: Air sac debris containing some fungal hyphae next to an embryonated *Serratospiculum* sp. egg. In some cases Serratospiculosis may trigger aspergillosis. PAS stain.

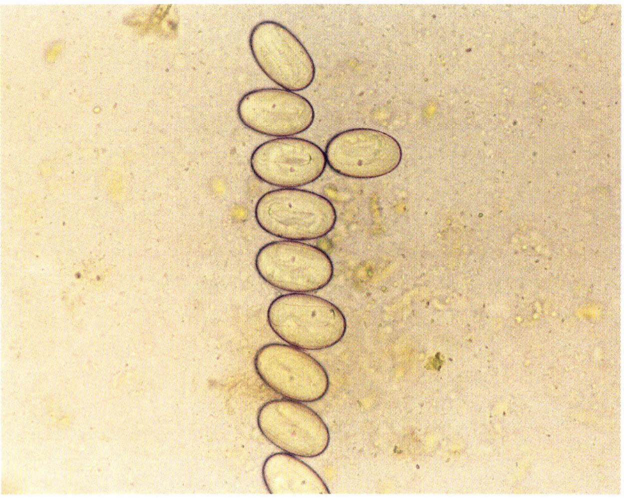

Figure 6.40: Large number of *Serratospiculum seurati* eggs in the faeces of a Saker falcon.

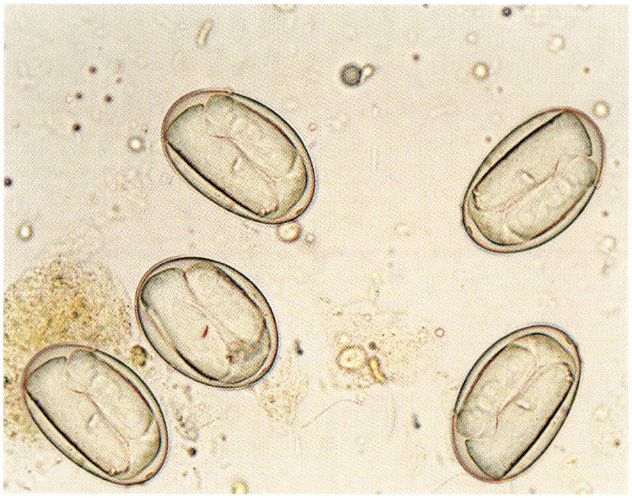

Figure 6.41: Five *Serratospiculum seurati* eggs in the faeces of a Saker falcon.

6

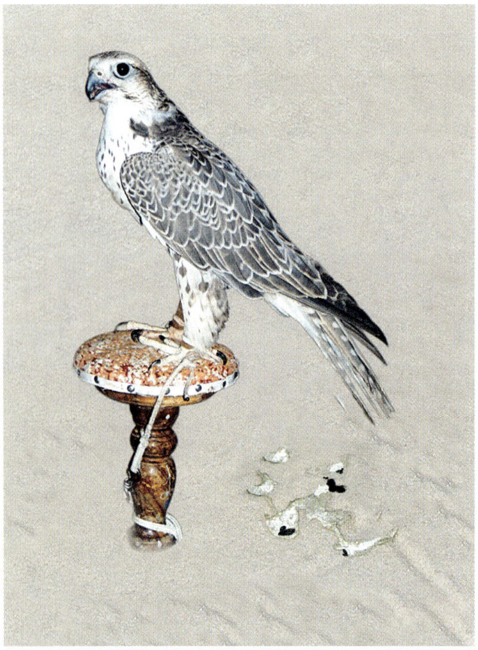

Figure 6.42: Falcons pass large amount of *Serratospiculum seurati* ova in the faeces.

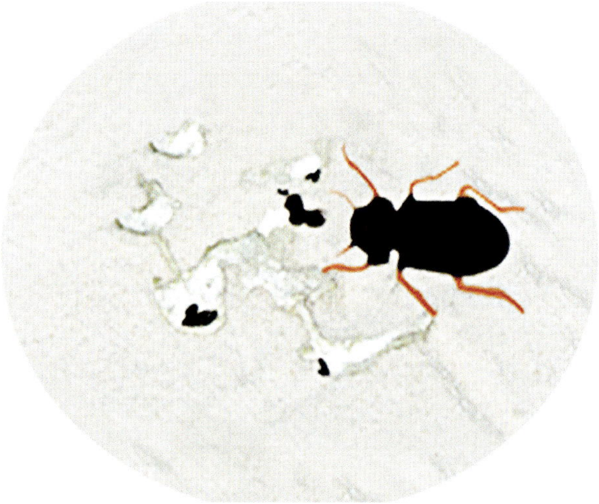

Figure 6.43: Some beetle species act as intermediary host during the development of the infective L3 larvae of *Serratospiculum seurati.*

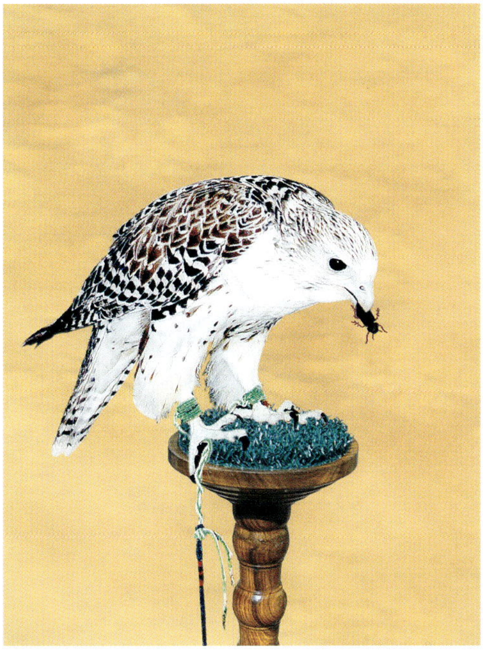

Figure 6.44: Falcons very commonly eat beetles roaming around the perches. This is the route in which the infective L3 larvae of *Serratospiculum seurati* is acquired by the final host.

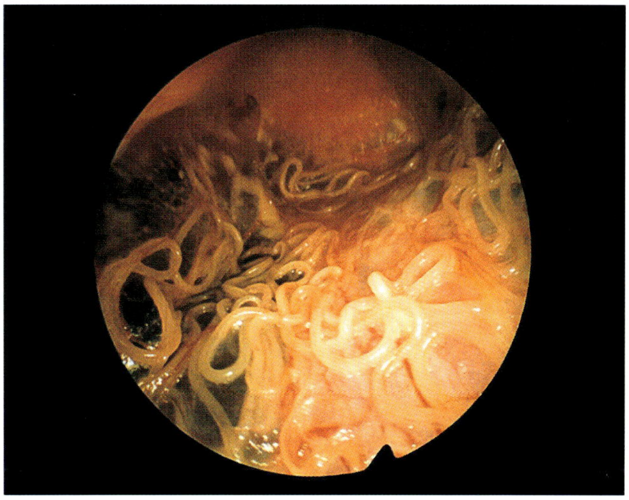

Figure 6.45: Endoscopic view of adult *Serratospiculum seurati* nematodes on the air sac walls of a Saker falcon.

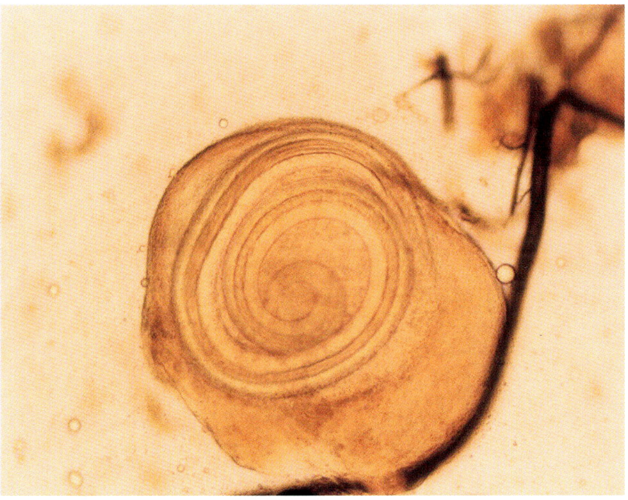

Figure 6.46: An embryonated L1 larva of *Serratospiculum seurati* obtained from the dissection of a beetle.

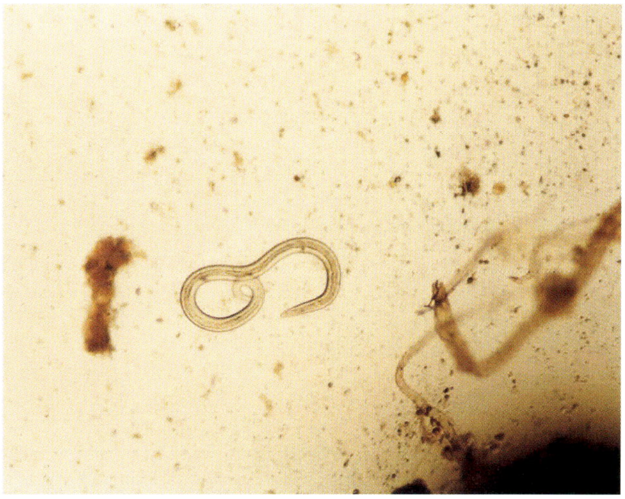

Figure 6.47: An L1 larva of *Serratospiculum seurati* from a beetle.

6

Capillariosis

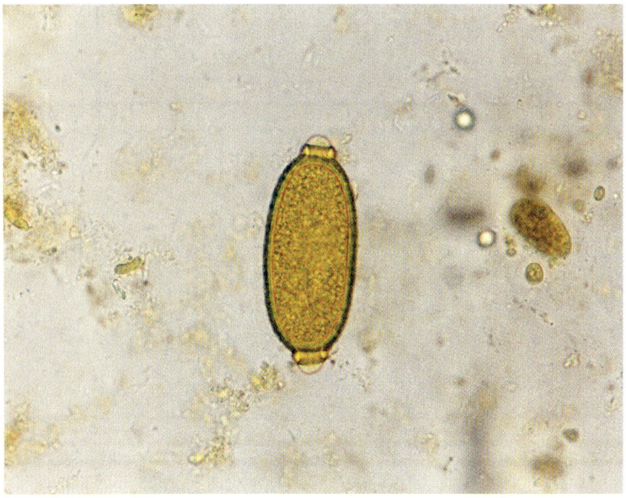

Figure 6.48: One *Capillaria* sp. egg in the faeces of a Saker falcon.

Trichinellosis

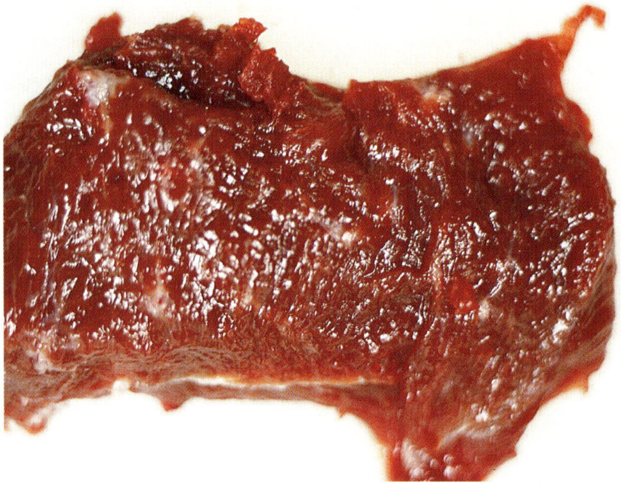

Figure 6.49: Pectoral muscle of a Saker falcon showing multiple submiliar, barely visible, grey spots in the deeper layers. Trichinellosis in raptors, caused by *Trichinella pseudospiralis*, is rare. The number of parasites and necrotic areas are higher in the pectoral muscle than in the leg muscles. The myocardium is usually free of parasites.

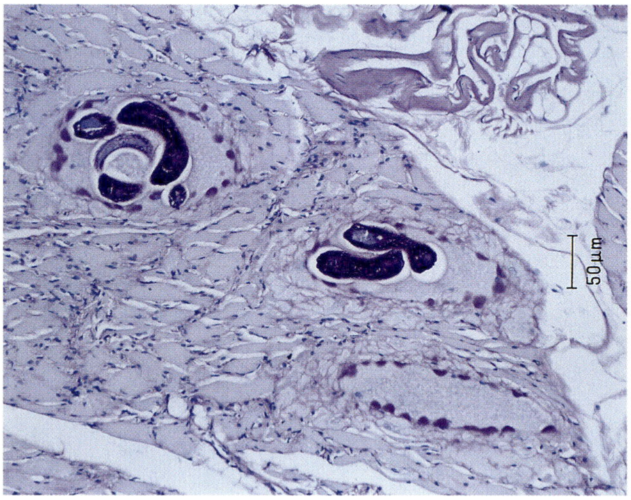

Figure 6.50: Muscle trichinellosis: Pectoral muscle of an Indian Peregrine falcon with two small coiled larvae within the sarcoplasma of the muscle fibers and a necrotic hyaline focus. In the proximity of the parasite, the attached fibers are swollen and pale with loss of myofibrils. These changes may have a negative effect on the performance of the falcon. *Trichinella pseudospiralis* does not develop a capsule, whereas *Trichinella spiralis* (mammalian parasite) is invariably surrounded by a capsule. HE stain.

Other helminths

Nematodes

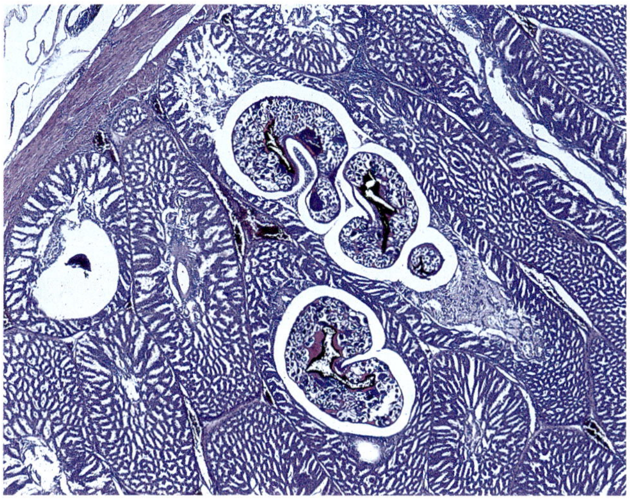

Figure 6.51: Proventriculus: Two nematodes located deep in the stomach gland complex with no associated inflammatory reaction. PAS stain.

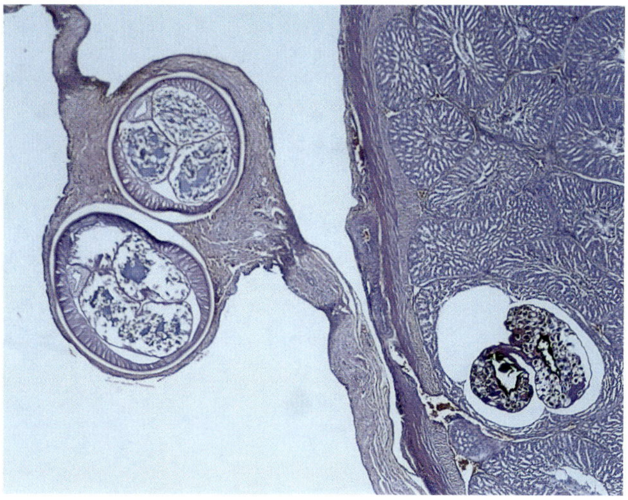

Figure 6.52: Proventriculus: Simultaneous *Spiruridae* spp. and *Serratospiculum* spp. infection. The nematode is deeply embedded in the stomach gland complex next to 2 *Serratospiculum* spp. parasites, which invaded in the serosa. PAS stain.

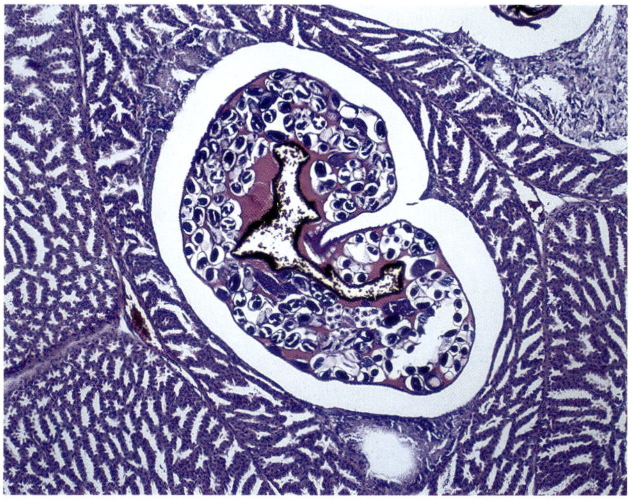

Figure 6.53: Higher magnification of Figure 6.52. The parasite is filled with numerous embryonated eggs. Size and shape are typical for *Spiruridae* spp. PAS stain.

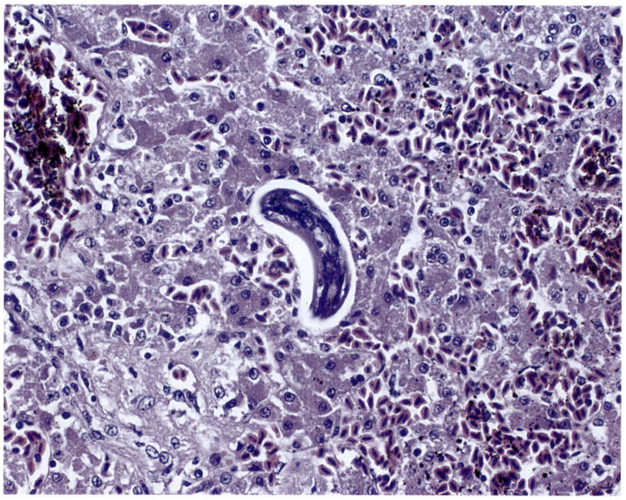

Figure 6.54: A small unidentified roundworm in the liver parenchyma of a Gyr falcon with no associated inflammatory reaction. PAS stain.

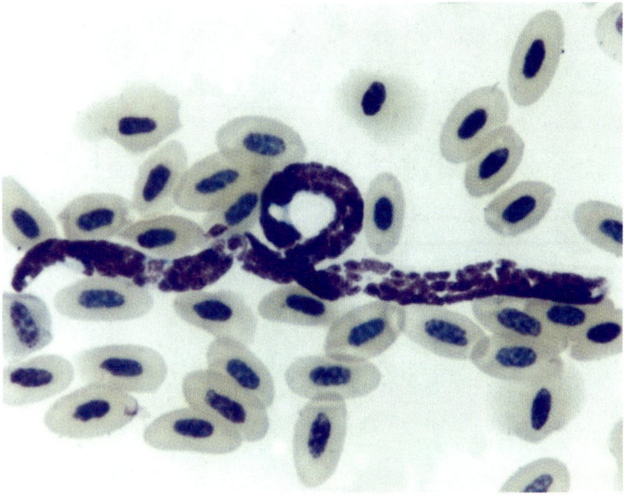

Figure 6.55: An unidentified microfilaria from a Saker falcon positioned between erythrocytes.

Anisakidae

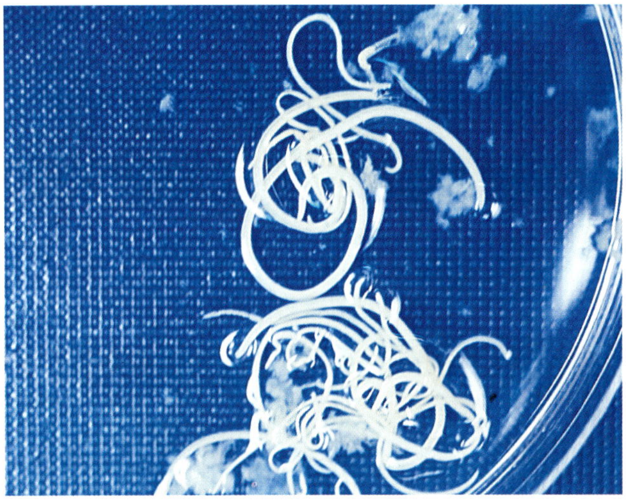

Figure 6.56: *Porrocaecum depressum* from a Saker falcon's small intestine.

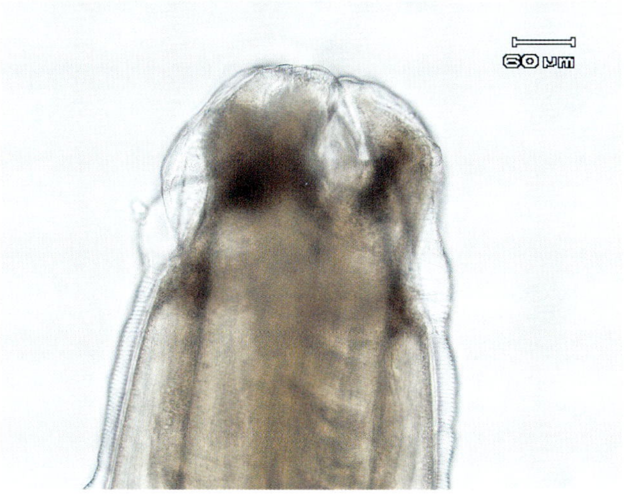

Figure 6.57 a: *Porrocaecum depressum* of a Peregrine falcon: Anterior end with free lips.

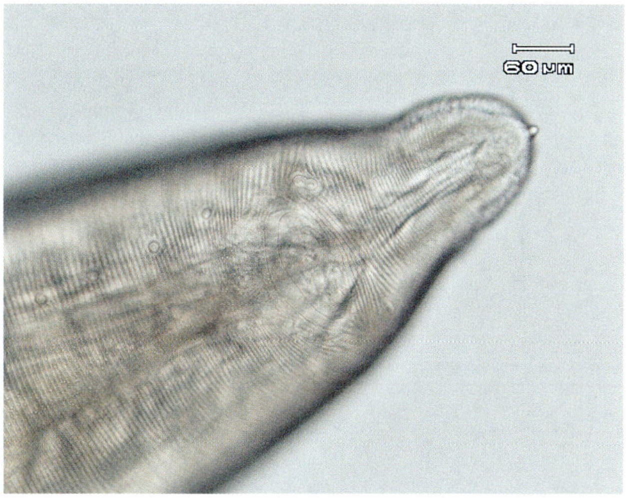

Figure 6.57 b: *Porrocaecum depressum* of a Peregrine falcon: Posterior end of a male showing the anal opening and pre and post-anal papillae.

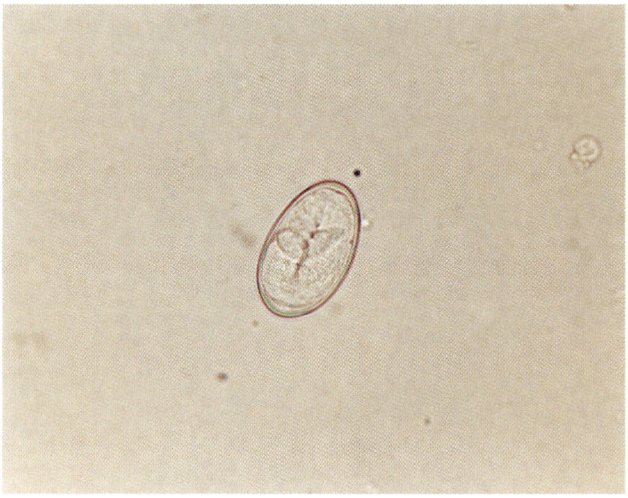

Figure 6.58: One *Paraspiralatus sakeri* egg in the faeces of a Saker falcon.

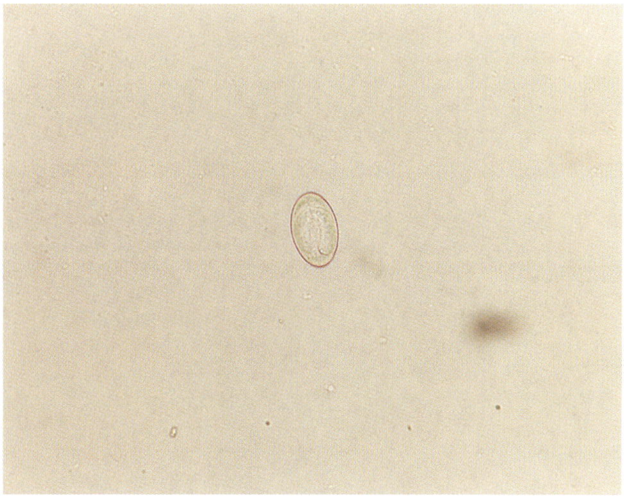

Figure 6.59: One *Physaloptera alata* egg in the faeces of a Saker falcon.

Cestodes (Tapeworms)

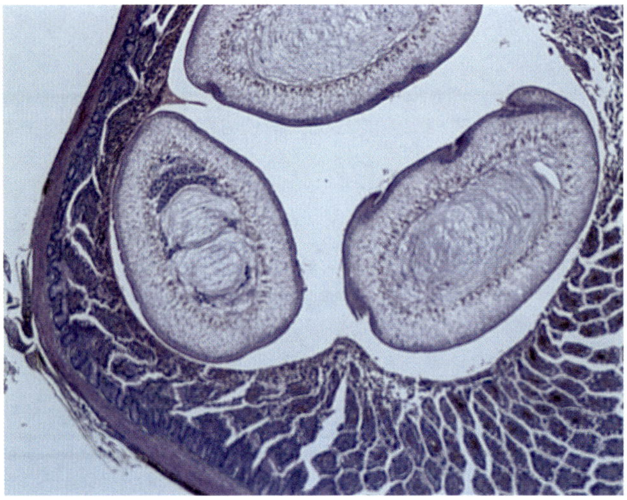

Figure 6.60: Three unidentified tape worms in the lumen of the small intestine of a Gyr falcon. HE stain.

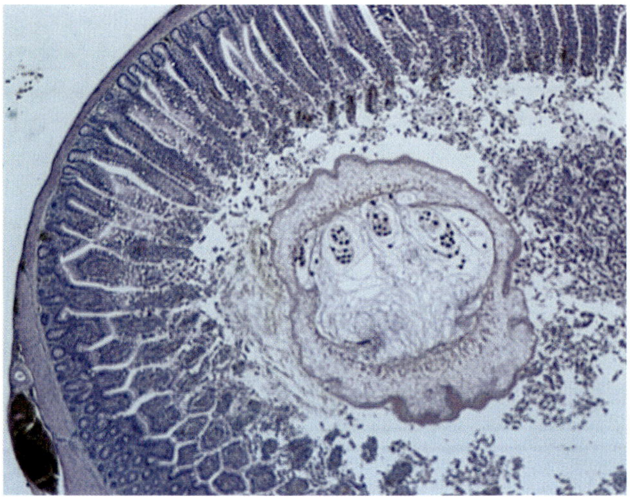

Figure 6.61: This picture shows the same tapeworm of Figure 6.60, but from a different location of the small intestine. These are segments of the uterus containing several eggs. HE stain.

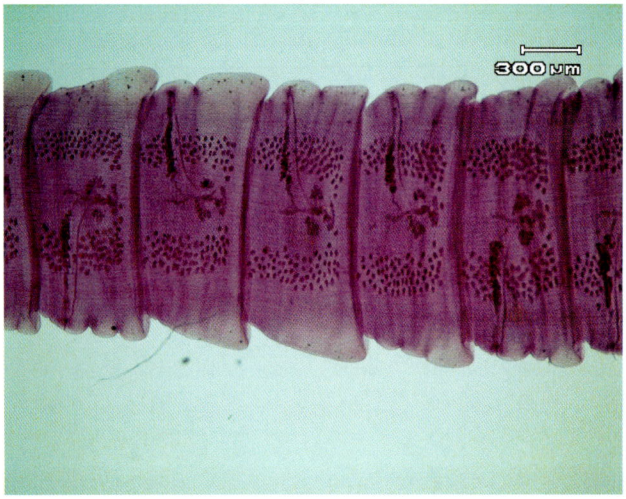

Figure 6.62: *Cladotaenia circi*, hermaphrodite segments. Numerous testes are grouped in two clusters laterally from the female reproductive organs. Genital pori alternate irregularly. Lactic acid carmin stain.

Trematodes (Flukes)

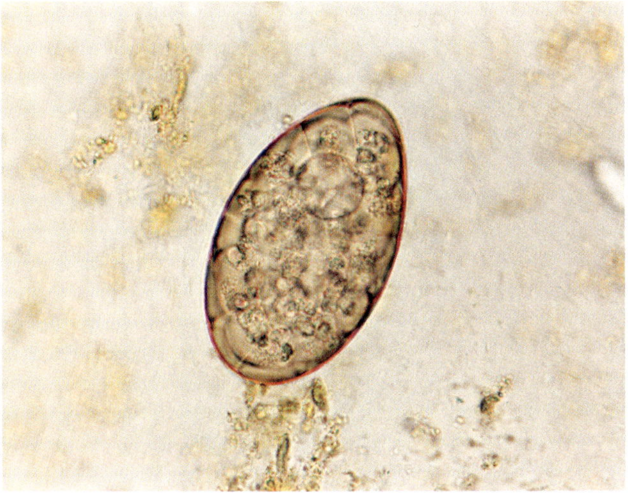

Figure 6.63: One *Strigea falconis* egg in the faeces of a Saker falcon.

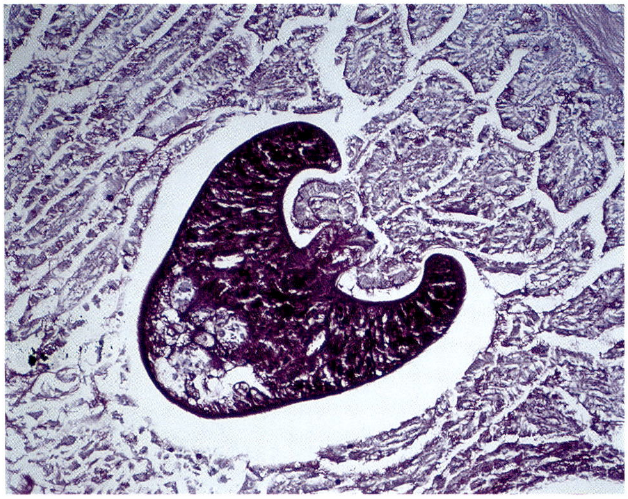

Figure 6.64: Trematode (transversal section) in the intestinal lumen of a Gyr x Peregrine hybrid. The parasite is located deep in the mucosa. PAS stain.

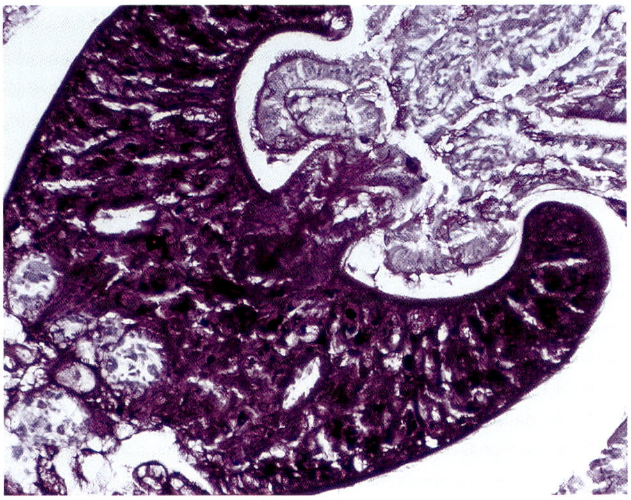

Figure 6.65: Higher magnification of Figure 6.64. The parasite is fixed at the mucosa with the tribozytic organ. This structure and the body shape are typical for *Strigeidae* spp. PAS stain.

Chapter 7

Miscellaneous Diseases

Poor performance

Bumblefoot

Amyloidosis

Gout

Lead intoxication

Ammonium chloride (schnather) intoxication

This chapter deals with poor performance, bumblefoot, metabolic diseases, lead and ammonium chloride intoxication. These diseases are quite common in hunting falcons and therefore haematology and biochemistry parameters are presented separately where possible. As can be clearly seen from the results, most of the diseases have little impact on haematology values but may result in significant alterations in biochemistry values.

Poor performance of hunting falcons has different causes. It can be caused by subclinical infections like chlamydophilosis, salmonella infection, mild coccidiosis or overtraining. Significant increase in CK, LDH, ALT, AST and GGT values are observed, indicating liver and muscle involvement. Iron is significantly decreased may be due to absorption difficulties in the duodenum and upper jejunum.

Amyloidosis is a life-threatening illness of hunting falcons, and seems to occur more often in Gyr falcons and Gyr hybrids. It is obviously seen in connection with chronic infections like aspergillosis, tuberculosis, chlamydophilosis, trichomonosis, bumblefoot and airsacculitis. BA, AST, ALT and GGT are significantly increased in cases of amyloidosis. In most amyloidosis falcons, a hyperglobinaemia is also observed.

Gout is a metabolic disorder primarily caused by kidney malfunction, and is usually associated with urinary tract disease, prolonged dehydration, exogenous stresses and nutritional disorders such as excessive intake of protein and calcium. In these cases, BUN and UA are high. However, pre-renal gout cases may die of gout having normal UA levels. These cases are often found in association with clostridial enterotoxaemia. In general very little is known about renal diseases in falcons and diagnosis is often speculative.

Lead toxicosis or plumbism is the most common heavy metal toxicity in captive falcons. It is caused when falcons ingest hidden shotgun pellets from pigeons or mammals that have been shot. Lead poisoning leads to hypochromic macrocytic anaemia and elevation of liver and kidney enzymes.

Ammonium chloride is an inorganic salt, commercially available as hygroscopic crystals or as a white crystalline powder. In the Middle East, ammonium chloride is best known as »Schnather« and routinely administered to falcons with the aim of improving their hunting ability. However, if the bird is not able to vomit the ingested crystal within 5 to 10 minutes, it will die due to the highly toxic agent.

Poor performance

Table 7.1: Haematology and biochemistry values of falcons suffering from poor performance

			Mean ± SD	
Parameters	SI Units	N	Diseased Falcons	Reference Values
RBC	$x10^{12}/\mu l$	123	3.10 ± 0.29	3.21 ± 0.30
HB	g/dl	123	14.67 ± 1.71	14.95 ± 1.39
HTC	l/l	123	0.44 ± 0.04	0.45 ± 0.04
MCV	fl	123	141.94 ± 8.63	139.85 ± 6.33
MCH	pg	123	47.32 ± 4.37	46.42 ± 2.55
WBC	$x10^{9}/l$	123	10.51 ± 4.93	9.64 ± 3.96
HETERO	%	123	58.30 ± 17.22	59.80 ± 12.87
LYMPHO	%	123	37.28 ± 6.01	34.84 ± 12.88
MONO	%	123	4.27 ± 1.11	4.46 ± 2.77
EOS	%	123	0.03	0.43
BASO	%	123	0.10	0.16
CK	U/L	191	▲ **1018** ± 97	640 ± 210
LDH	U/L	191	▲ **1398** ± 311	1028 ± 385
ALT	U/L	191	▲ **123.02** ± 40.10	64.8 ± 28.9
AST	U/L	191	▲ **148.18** ± 10.22	93.1 ± 44.6
GGT	U/L	191	▲ **18.3** ± 7.4	14.0 ± 6.3
BUN	mmol/l	127	5.1 ± 1.9	4.7 ± 1.8
UA	µmol/l	91	547 ± 311	487 ± 267
BA	µmol/l	160	21.5 ± 3.9	22.3 ± 4.7
TP	g/l	41	26.7 ± 5.4	28.4 ± 6.5
ALB	g/l	41	10.1 ± 1.0	10.4 ± 1.9
GLOB	g/l	41	16.6 ± 4.5	18.0 ± 4.6
IRON	µmol/l	92	▼ **3.6** ± 1.7	6.1 ± 3.7
CA	mmol/l	41	2.2 ± 0.4	2.4 ± 0.3
PHOS	mmol/l	36	0.8 ± 0.4	0.7 ± 0.3

Bumblefoot

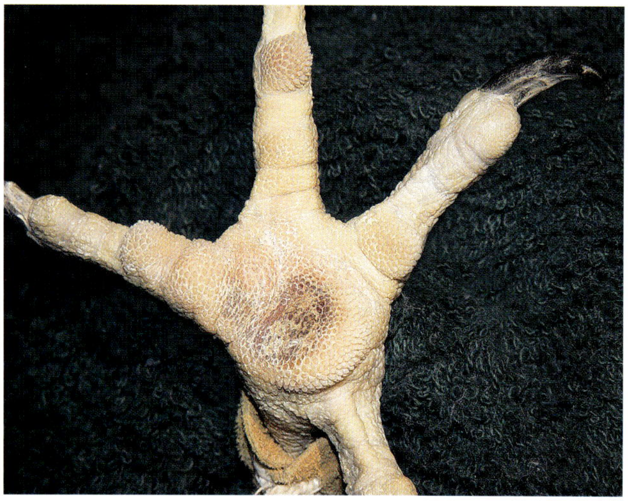

Figure 7.1: A mild form of bumblefoot.

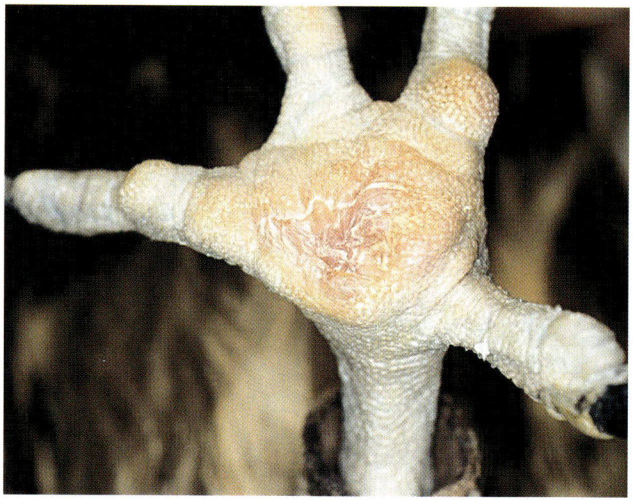

Figure 7.2: A medium severe case of bumblefoot.

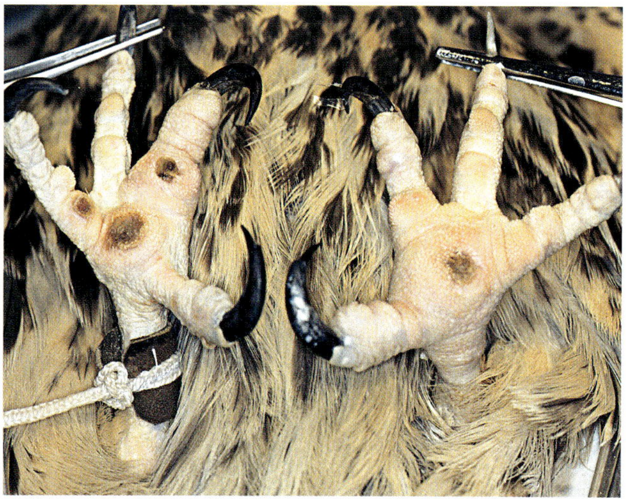

Figure 7.3: Bumblefoot begins with a dark thickened area in the centre of the sole of the feet. This is the result of the accumulation of dead cells, debris, blood and other fluids.

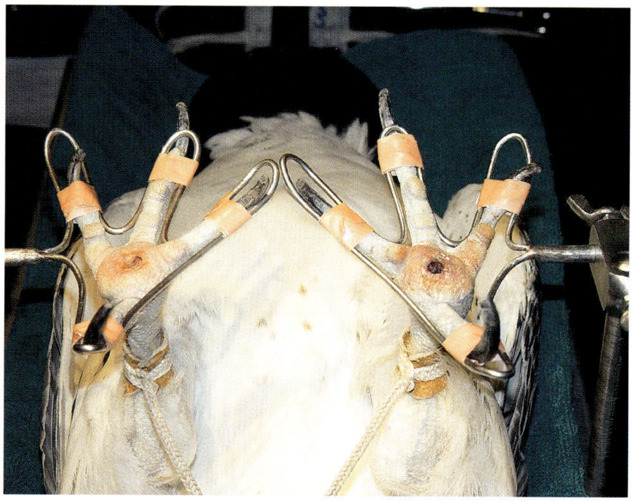

Figure 7.4: Most severe case of bumblefoot must be corrected surgically.

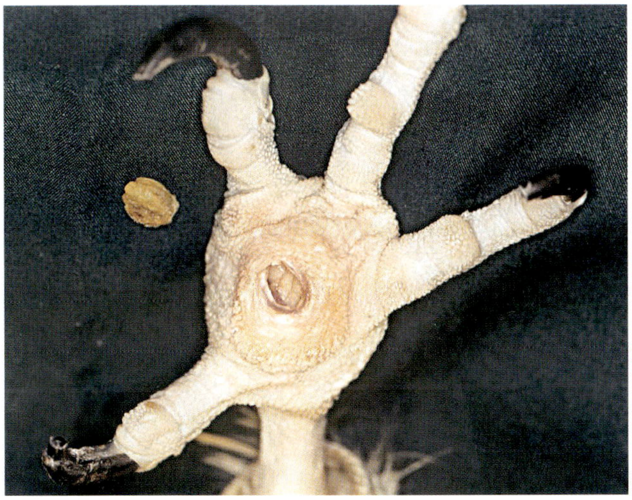

Figure 7.5: The scab on the central plantar surface is removed. Skin edges should be debrided and closed with a suitable suture material.

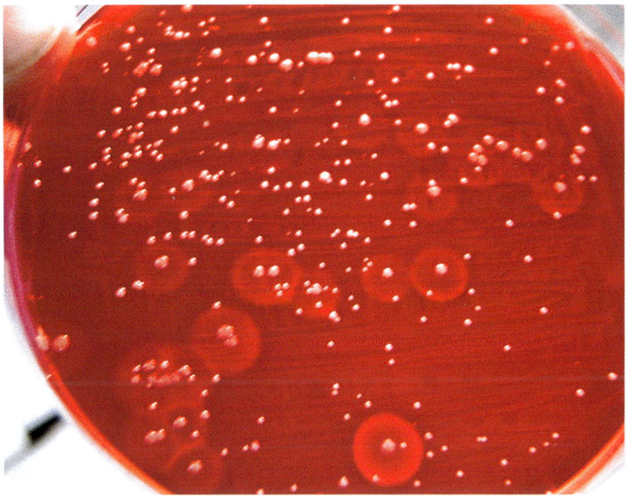

Figure 7.6: Growth of *Staphylococcus aureus* on blood agar. In over 90 % of bumblefoot cases, *Staphylococcus aureus* is isolated.

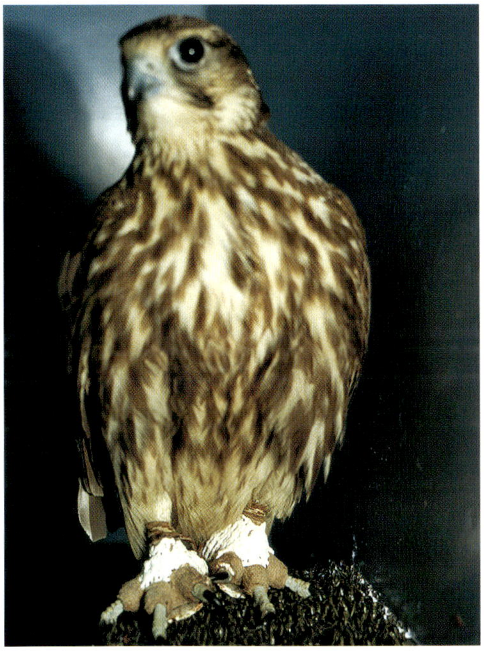

Figure 7.7: This Saker falcon, which suffered from bilateral bumblefoot, is standing on a specially designed cast to reduce focal pressure on the lesions. Different casting methods have been established to provide comfort to the bird following surgical treatment.

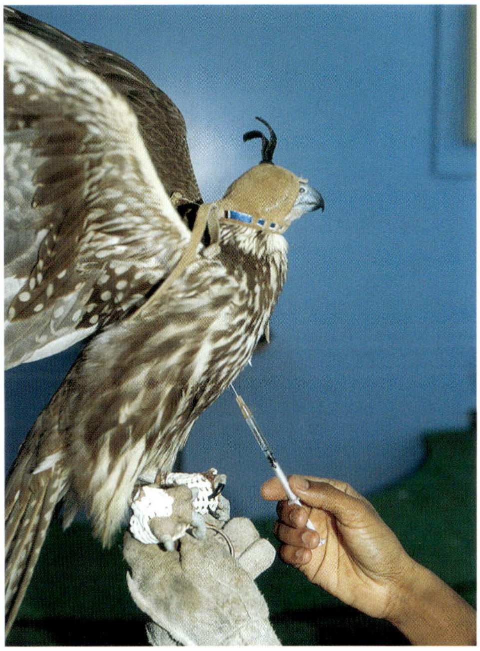

Figure 7.8: Antibiotic treatment is essential for the healing of bumblefoot. It is recommended that an antimicrobial sensitivity test is performed on the bacterial species isolated.

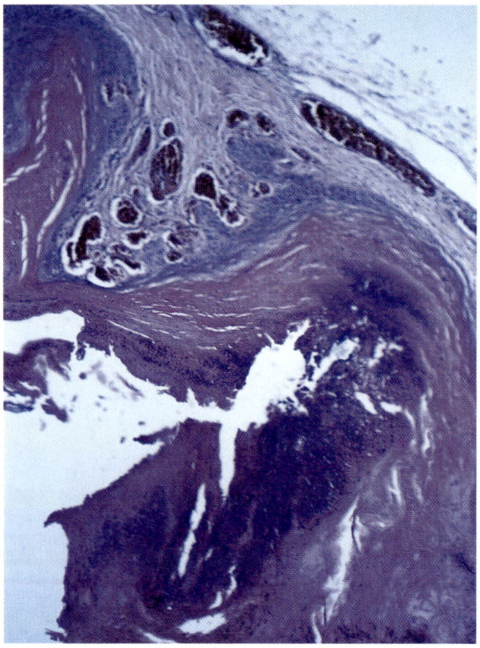

Figure 7.9: Severe pododermatitis with hyperkeratosis and extensive necroses, secondarily infected with bacteria. Gyr hybrid with severe bumblefoot. HE stain.

7

Amyloidosis

Table 7.2: Haematology and biochemistry values of 18 falcons suffering from amyloidosis

Para-meters	SI Units	Mean ± SD Diseased Falcons	Reference Values
RBC	$x10^{12}/\mu l$	3.18 ± 0.34	3.21 ± 0.30
HB	g/dl	14.67 ± 1.53	14.95 ± 1.39
HCT	l/l	0.44 ± 0.05	0.45 ± 0.04
MCV	fl	138.36 ± 8.00	139.85 ± 6.33
MCH	pg	46.13 ± 2.93	46.42 ± 2.55
WBC	$x10^9/l$	▲ **11.42** ± 3.03	9.64 ± 3.96
HETERO	%	60.54 ± 21.93	59.80 ± 12.87
LYMPHO	%	33.14 ± 11.82	34.84 ± 12.88
MONO	%	6.21 ± 1.10	4.46 ± 2.77
EOS	%	0.07	0.43
BASO	%	0.04	0.16
CK	U/L	▼ **512** ± 140	640 ± 210
LDH	U/L	nd *	1028 ± 385
ALT	U/L	▲ **186.4** ± 71.3	64.8 ± 28.9
AST	U/L	▲ **199.4** ± 84.8	93.1 ± 44.6
GGT	U/L	▲ **115.3** ± 7.1	14.0 ± 6.3
BUN	mmol/l	▲ **6.7** ± 2.6	4.7 ± 1.8
UA	µmol/l	470 ± 195	487 ± 267
BA	µmol/l	▲ **200**	22.3 ± 4.7
TP	g/l	▲ **39.3** ± 11.4	28.4 ± 6.5
ALB	g/l	11.6 ± 1.0	10.4 ± 1.9
GLOB	g/l	▲ **27.7** ± 10.4	18.0 ± 4.6
IRON	µmol/l	▲ **8.3** ± 0.5	6.1 ± 3.7
CA	mmol/c	2.6 ± 0.2	2.4 ± 0.3
PHOS	mmol/l	0.8 ± 0.4	0.7 ± 0.3

* nd = not done

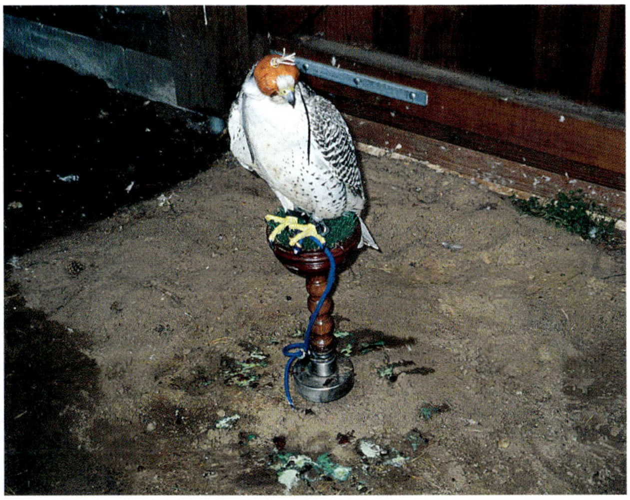

Figure 7.10: A Gyr falcon suffering from fatal amyloidosis. In terminal stages, green mutes are released due to the destruction of the liver parenchyma. These signs may be confused with inclusion body hepatitis (herpes). Like this falcon, falcons with amyloidosis can be in excellent body condition.

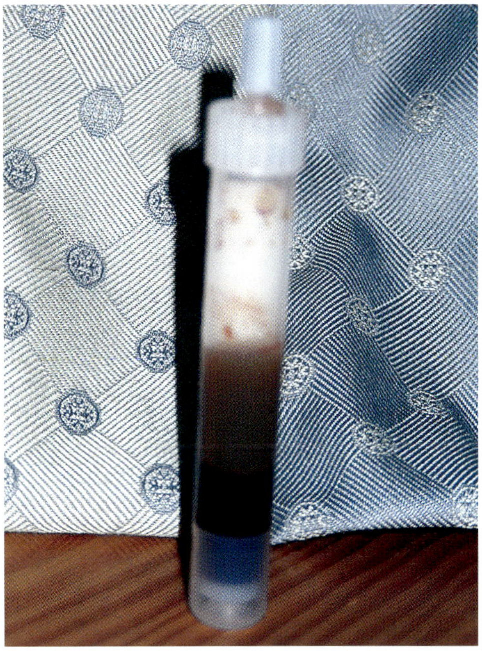

Figure 7.11: A blood sample from a Gyr falcon with fatal amyloidosis. The blood was centrifuged showing a brownish-grey serum. The colour is caused by the destruction of the liver parenchyma, releasing bile into the circulatory system.

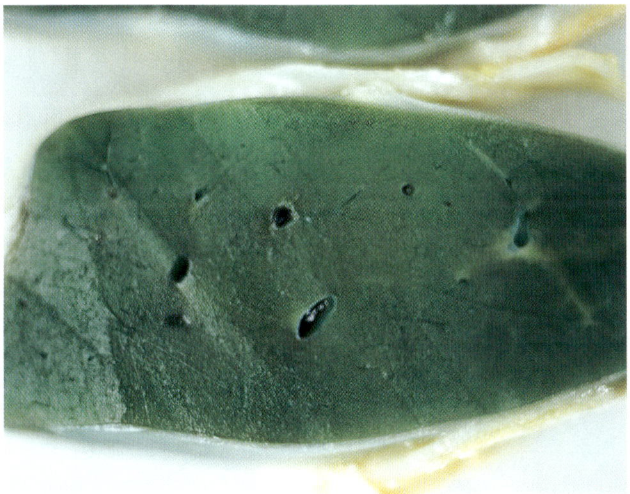

Figure 7.12: Liver of a Gyr falcon with amyloidosis which exhibits a greenish-brown colour; the liver is enlarged and firm.

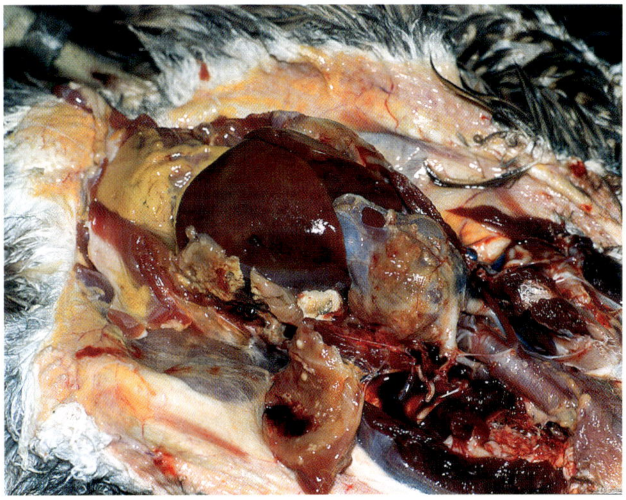

Figure 7.13: A female Peregrine falcon with amyloidosis. The liver is enlarged and brown-yellowish. The right caudal airsac is opened and exhibits whitish fungal Aspergillus granulomas. Chronic aspergillosis has predisposed to the development of amyloidosis. Due to the grave prognosis this bird was euthanized.

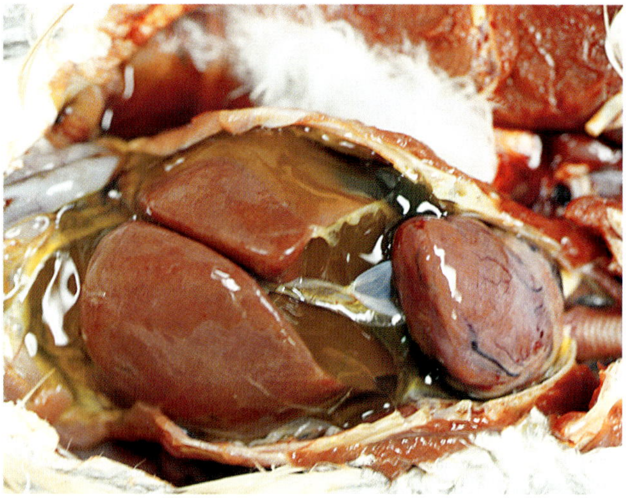

Figure 7.14: A female Gyr falcon with amyloidosis. Massive hepatomegaly with severe exudation on the serosa.

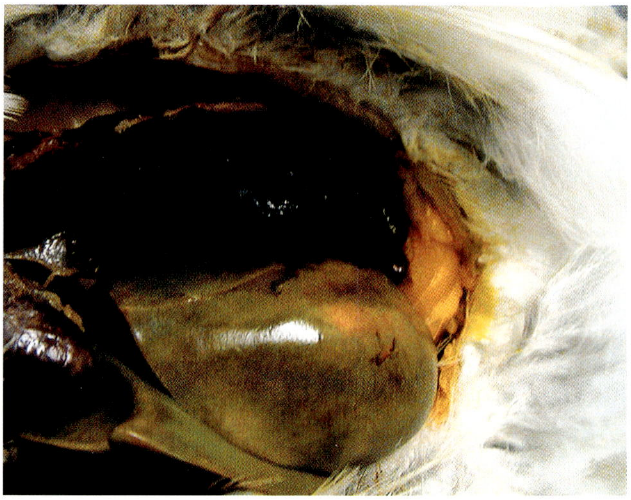

Figure 7.15: Liver rupture caused by amyloidosis in a male Gyr falcon with a large quantity of coagulated blood attached to the liver.

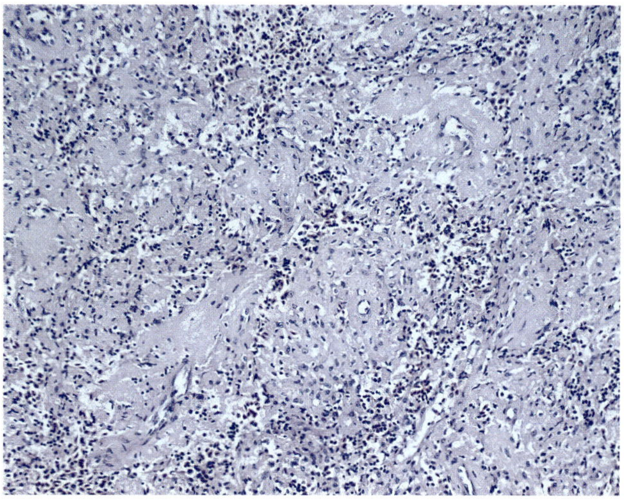

Figure 7.16: Amyloidosis of the spleen of a Gyr hybrid: Large amyloid-deposits mainly around large vessels causing depletion of the parenchyma. The spleen is involved in most cases of amyloidosis. HE stain.

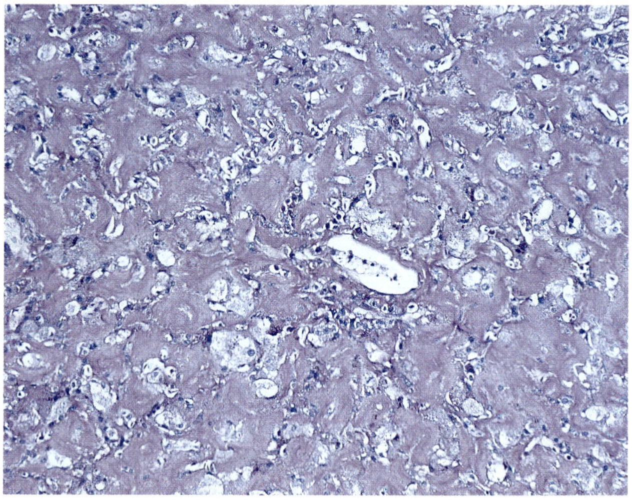

Figure 7.17: Massive amyloid-deposits in the Disse space of a Gyr hybrid causing atrophy of the liver parenchyma resulting in dysfunction (green mute). As in other avians most probably AA-amyloid is involved in falcon amyloidosis. PAS stain.

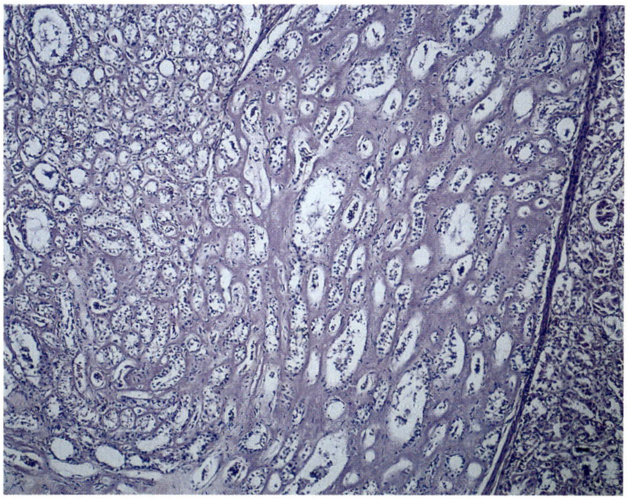

Figure 7.18: Amyloidosis of a Gyr's kidney: Amyloid deposits in the medullary interstitium. Glomerular deposits are rarely seen in falcons. Amyloid can be visualised also by Thioflavin or Congo red staining. PAS stain.

Gout

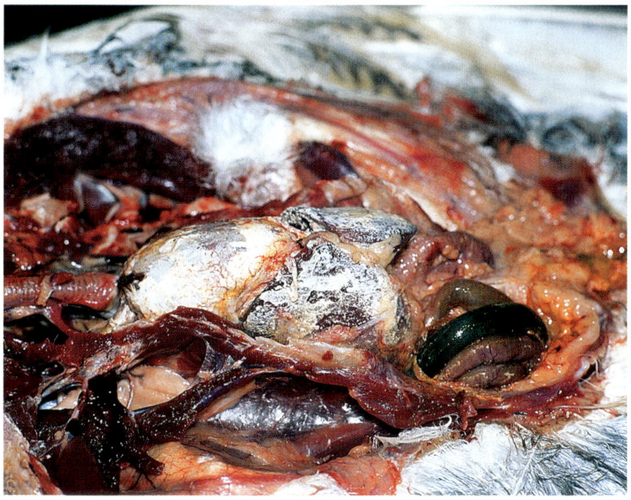

Figure 7.19: Visceral gout of a Gyr falcon. After the long and hot summer season, an increased number of falcons regularly die in the Middle East from visceral gout. It is likely that the disease is triggered by prolonged dehydration. BUN and UA values in this bird were 10.1 mmol/l and 812 µmol/l, respectively.

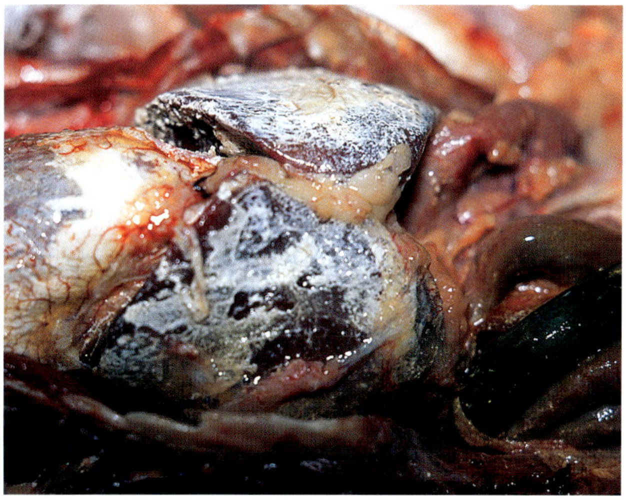

Figure 7.20: A close-up of the same falcon as in Figure 7.19.

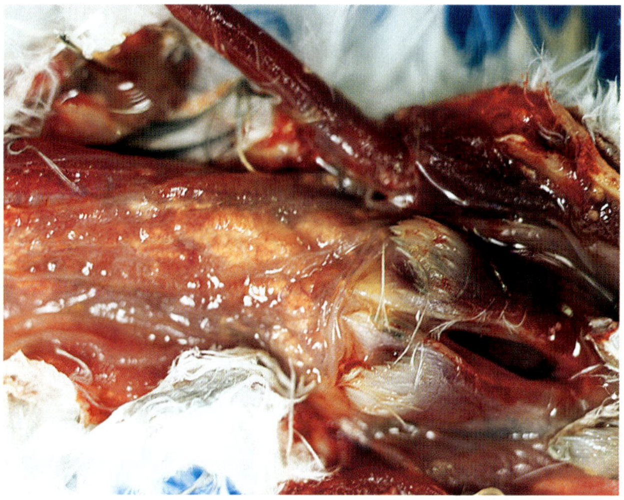

Figure 7.21: Whitish deposits in the oesophageal mucosa. In cases of visceral gout, urate deposits can be found within or on the surface of any organs.

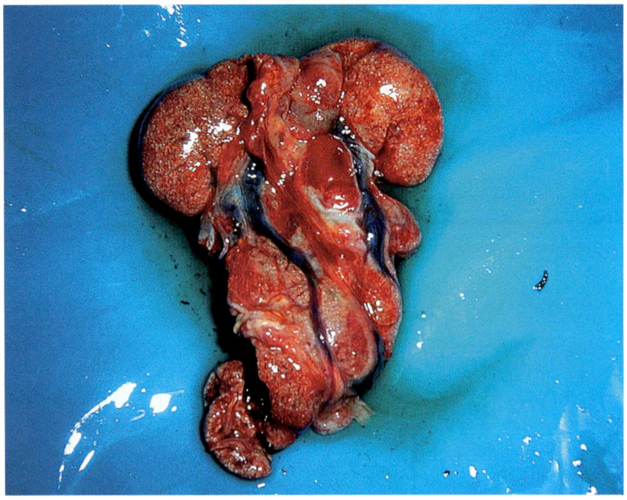

Figure 7.22: Swollen kidneys of a Gyr falcon with the typical miliar white spots in the parenchyma, a finding which is pathognomic for gout.

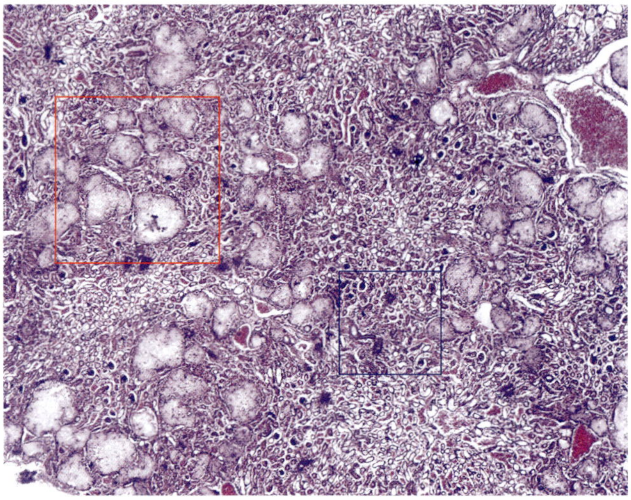

Figure 7.23: Renal gout: Multifocal renal tubular necrosis with large pale necrotic foci (highlighted in red) (typical for water deprivation) and numerous small dark urate deposits (highlighted in blue). At least in falcons in the Middle East, water deprivation seems to be a major cause of gout despite water being readily available. HE stain.

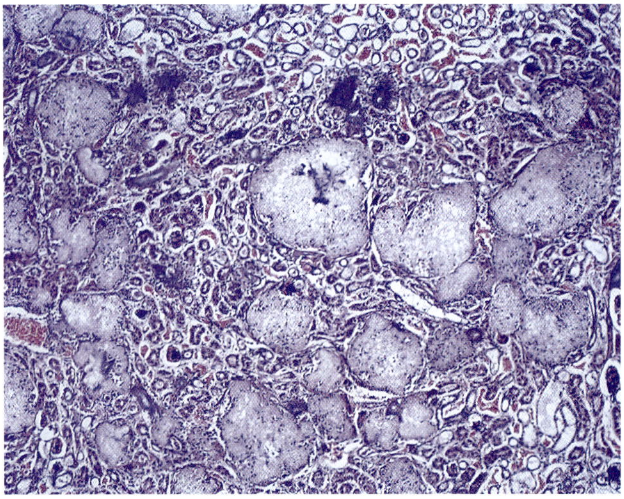

Figure 7.24: Higher magnification of Figure 7.23 showing extensive tubular necrosis surrounded by urate deposits. HE stain.

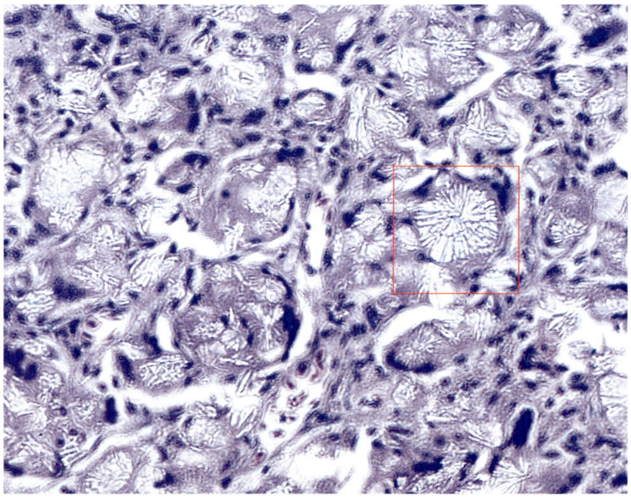

Figure 7.25: Airsac gout: Numerous urate crystals with central radiation surrounded by macrophages forming granulomas. Urate crystals are easy dissolved in formalin. In this case, poor penetration of the formalin resulted in preservation of urate-crystals in the tissue. HE stain.

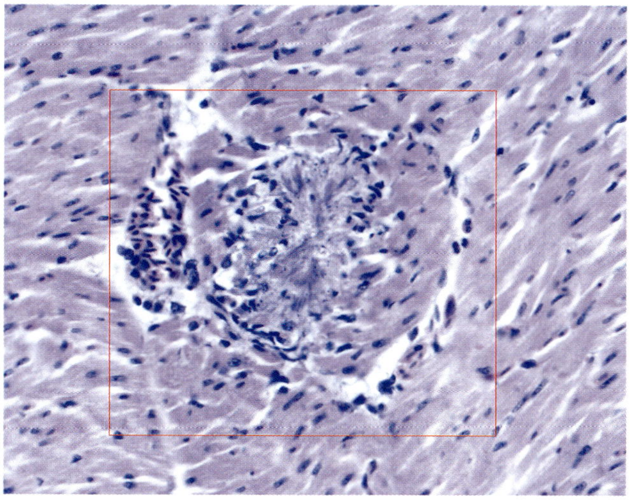

Figure 7.26: Gout of the heart: Urate deposits within the myocardium of a Gyr x Peregrine hybrid causing granulomatous lesions. The urate crystals have disappeared during formalin fixation. However, the original shape of the previously present crystals is still visible. HE stain.

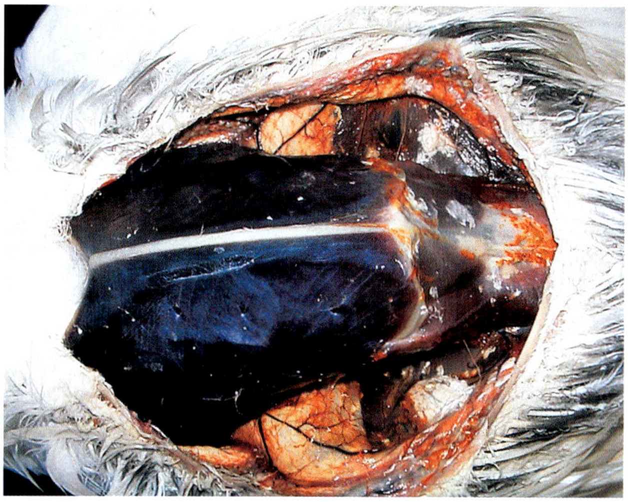

Figure 7.27: Subcutaneous gout indicated by white deposits on the abdominal muscle of a Gyr falcon.

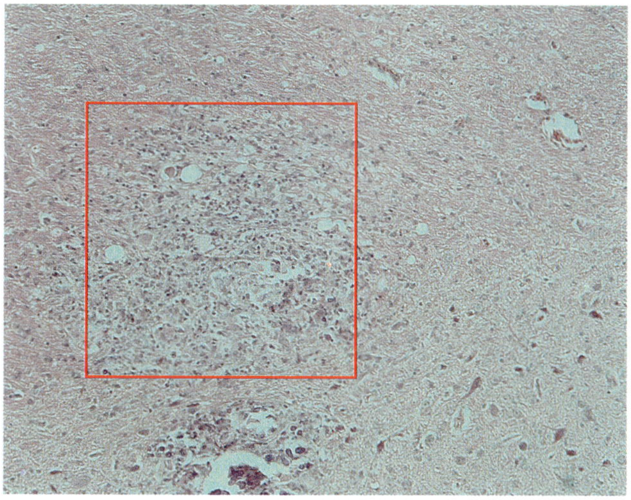

Figure 7.28: Granulomatous encephalitis in a Gyr falcon caused by urate deposits.

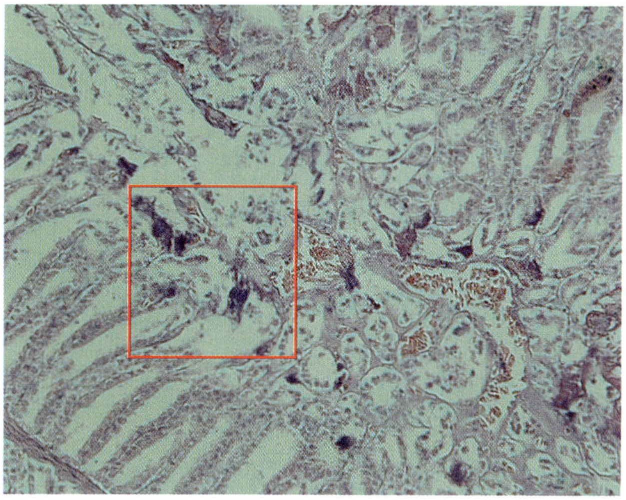

Figure 7.29: Diffuse urate deposits in the proventriculus gland of a Gyr falcon.

Lead intoxication

Table 7.3: Haematology and biochemistry values of falcons suffering from lead intoxication

Parameters	SI Units	N	Mean ± SD Diseased Falcons	Reference Values
RBC	$x10^{12}/l$	29	▼ **2.74** ± 0.34	3.21 ± 0.30
HB	g/dl	29	▼ **13.00** ± 1.80	14.95 ± 1.39
HCT	l/l	29	▼ **0.39** ± 0.05	0.45 ± 0.04
MCV	fl	29	▲ **142.34** ± 5.38	139.85 ± 6.33
MCH	pg	29	▲ **47.45** ± 2.43	46.42 ± 2.55
WBC	$x10^{9}/l$	27	▲ **13.61** ± 4.51	9.64 ± 3.96
HETERO	%	28	60.36 ± 16.81	59.80 ± 12.87
LYMPHO	%	28	35.71 ± 15.99	34.84 ± 12.88
MONO	%	28	3.93 ± 3.83	4.46 ± 2.77
EOS	%	28	0.00	0.43
BASO	%	28	0.00	0.16
CK	U/L	22	▲ **805** ± 167	640 ± 210
LDH	U/L	26	970 ± 101	1028 ± 385
ALT	U/L	26	▲ **223.7** ± 34.1	64.8 ± 28.9
AST	U/L	26	▲ **155.3** ± 30.5	93.1 ± 44.6
GGT	U/L	22	15.8 ± 7.6	14.0 ± 6.3
BUN	mmol/l	13	5.1 ± 1.8	4.7 ± 1.8
UA	µmol/l	19	▲ **611** ± 89	487 ± 267
BA	µmol/l	25	21.5 ± 3.9	22.3 ± 4.7
TP	g/l	29	30.8 ± 5.2	28.4 ± 6.5
ALB	g/l	29	12.9 ± 2.3	10.4 ± 1.9
GLOB	g/l	29	17.9 ± 3.7	18.0 ± 4.6
IRON	µmol/l	23	▼ **3.1** ± 7.9	6.1 ± 3.7
CA	mmol	23	2.9 ± 0.4	2.4 ± 0.3
PHOS	mmol/l	25	▲ **1.2** ± 0.6	0.7 ± 0.3

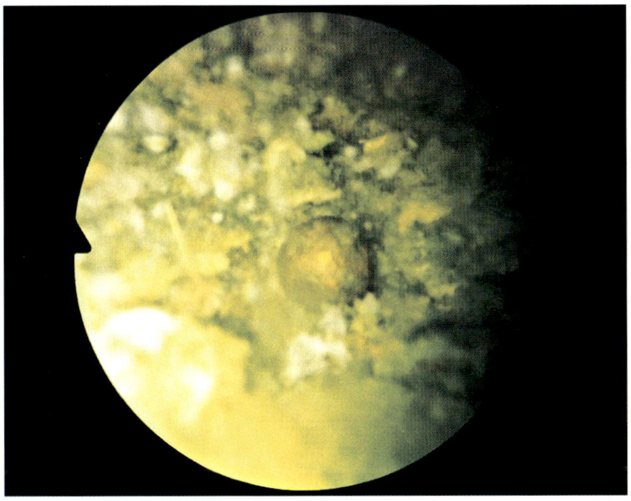

Figure 7.30: Lead pellets present in the stomach are removed by a combination of gastric lavage and retrieval using flexible or rigid endoscopes and long grasping forceps.

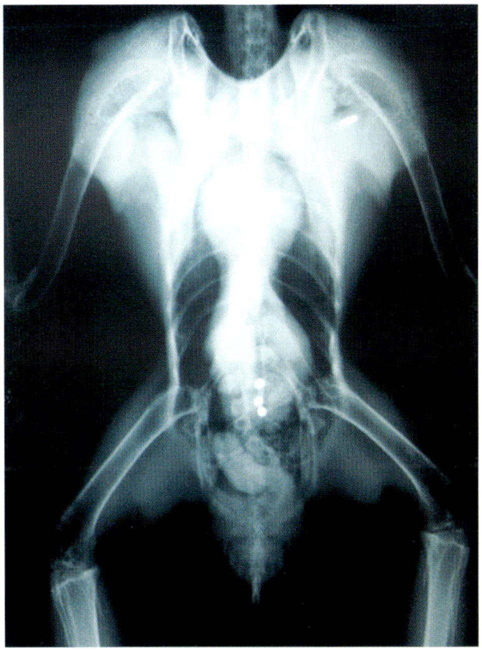

Figure 7.31: The diagnosis of lead toxicosis is usually carried out through radiology and by measuring the lead level in blood samples.

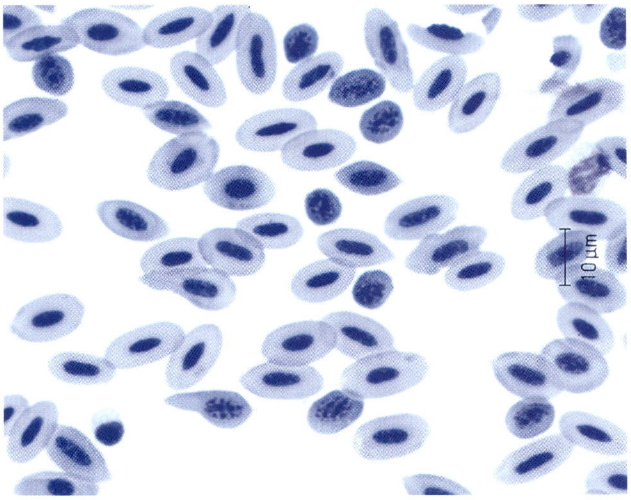

Figure 7.32: Hypochromic anaemia as well as hypochromasia, anisocytosis, microcytosis and poikilocytosis of a Saker falcon with lead intoxication (HB 8.6 g/dl).

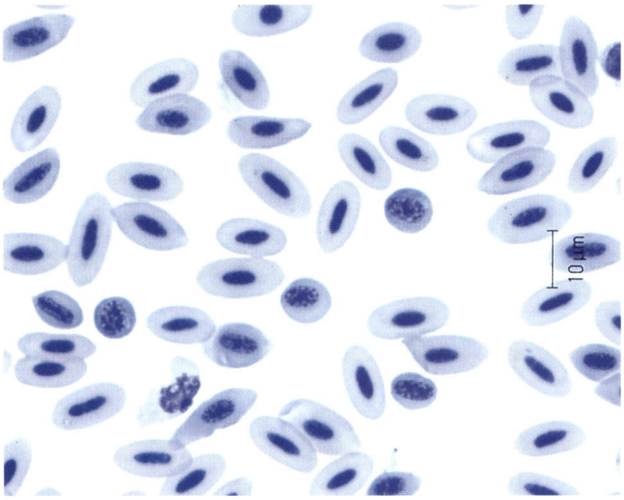

Figure 7.33: Lead poisoning of a Gyr hybrid. This falcon showed a liver lead level of 85.5 µg/dl. In falcons, liver lead levels of less than 40 µg/dl are normal. This falcon developed a hypochromic regenerative anaemia. Its HB value was 9.2 g/dl.

Ammonium chloride (schnather) intoxication

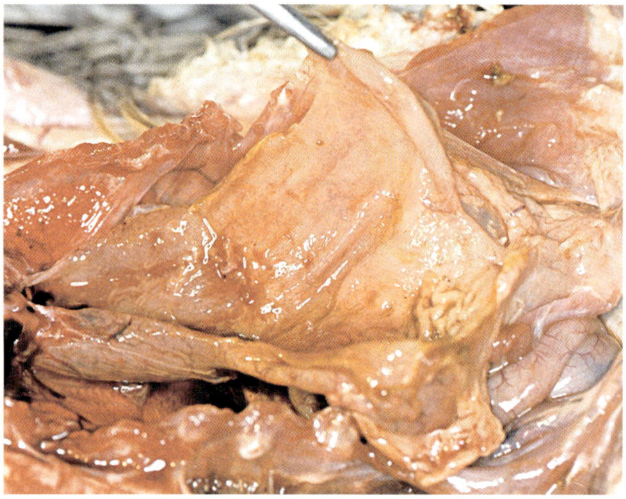

Figure 7.34: Stomach lining of a clinically normal Saker falcon. Note the healthy pink appearance of the mucosa.

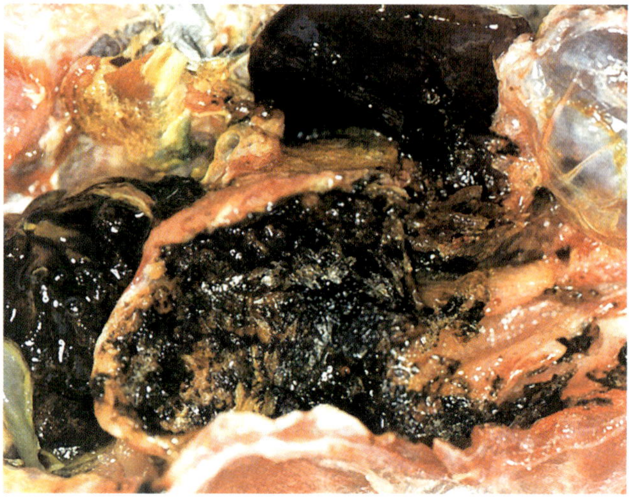

Figure 7.35: Stomach lining of a falcon that died of ammonium chloride toxicosis. Note the severe congestion and multiple haemorrhages of the mucosa.

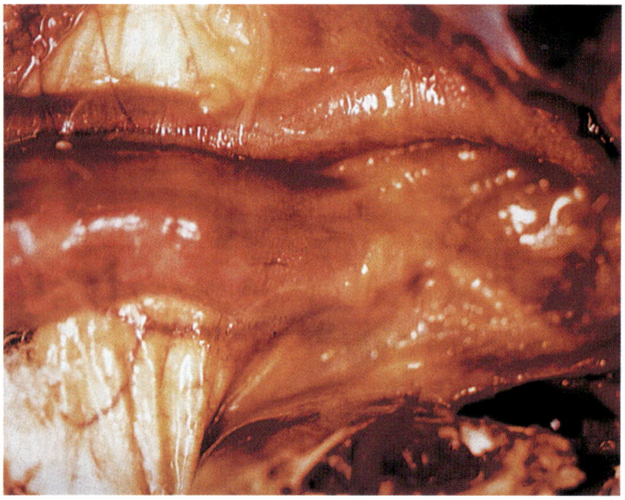

Figure 7.36: Crop of a Peregrine falcon with a very thin transparent mucosa with ammonium chloride toxicosis. HE stain.

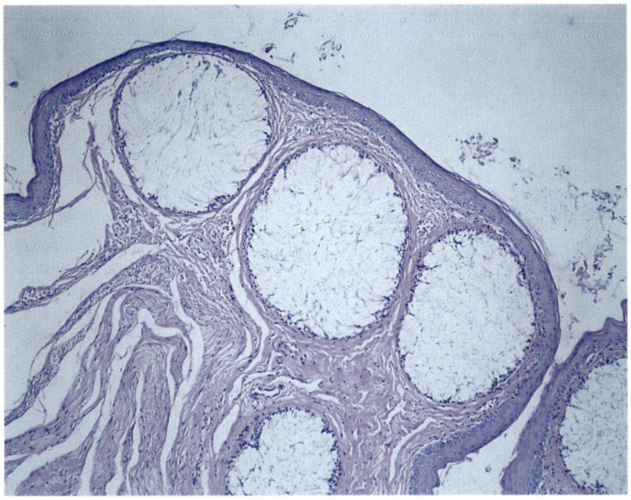

Figure 7.37 a: Thin epithelium of a crop of a Saker falcon consisting of only few layers of cells without keratinisation; no inflammation seen. The activated crop glands show hypersecretion. The thin crop epithelium is a sign of ammonium chloride intoxication. HE stain.

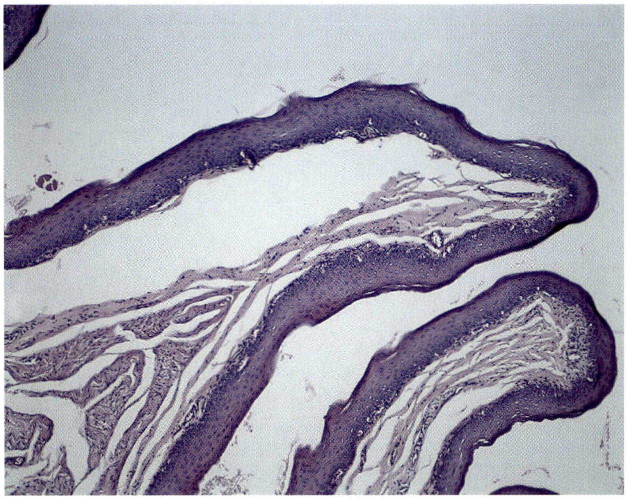

Figure 7.37 b: Crop epithelium of a clinically normal Peregrine falcon. HE stain.

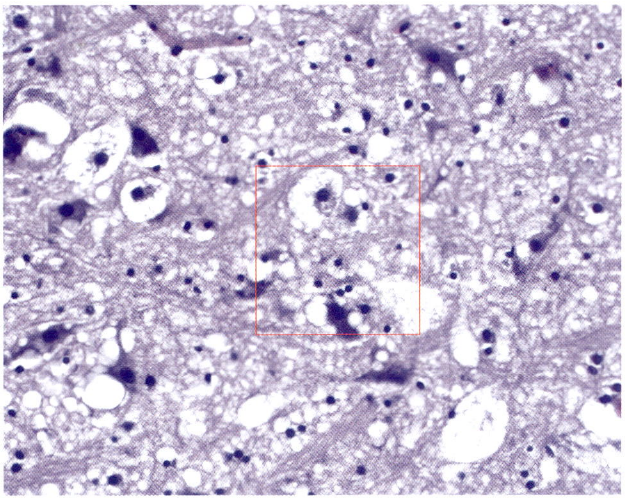

Figure 7.38: This picture shows the neurotoxic effects of the drug in a Saker falcon: Marked perineuronal oedema and gliosis. Toxicological analysis of this case revealed an ammonium chloride content of 3 mg per g intestinal content. HE stain.

Chapter 8

Diseases of Unknown Aetiology

Brain

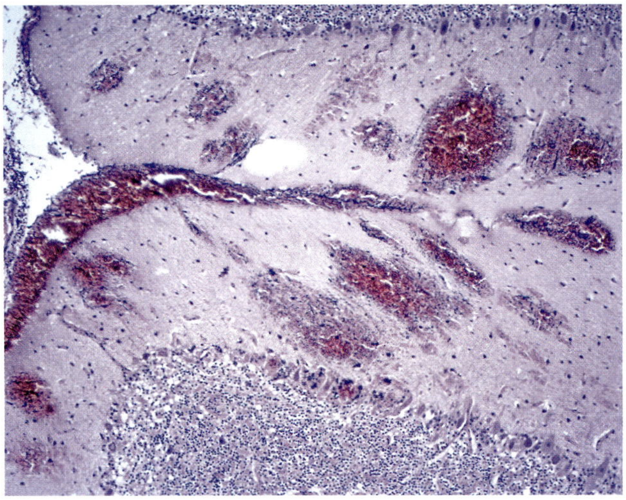

Figure 8.1: Brain, cerebellum. Massive meningeal and cerebellar haemorrhages in a Gyr x Peregrine hybrid, most probably after injury. HE stain.

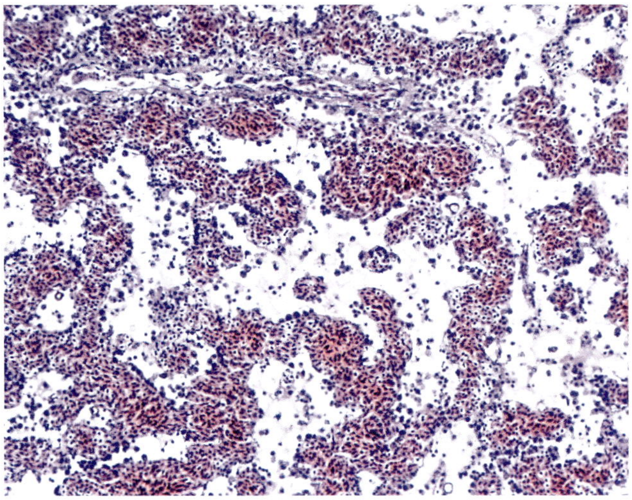

Figure 8.2: Higher magnification of Figure 8.1 with numerous small acute cerebellar haemorrhages next to large vessel. This concussion was the cause of death in this case. HE stain.

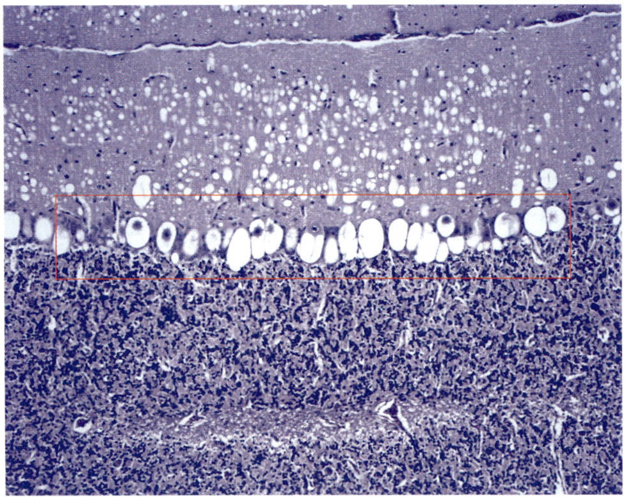

Figure 8.3: Brain, cerebellum. Neuronal vacuolar degeneration of unknown reason in a Gyr falcon, showing central-nervous signs. HE stain.

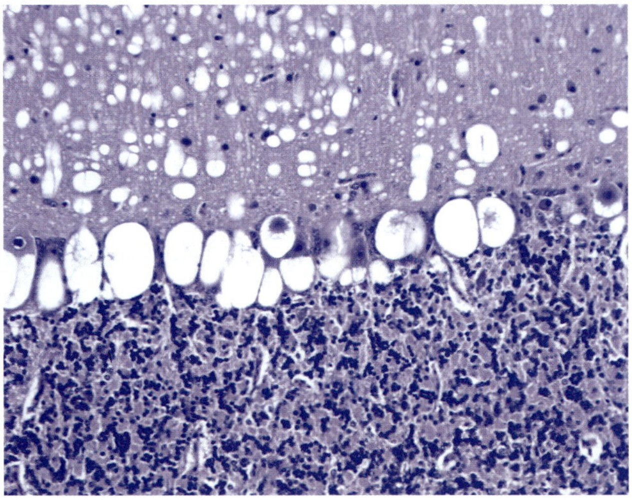

Figure 8.4: Higher magnification of Figure 8.3. Most of the Purkinje cells are degenerated leaving just empty cells. There is no inflammatory reaction around these cells. HE stain.

Muscle

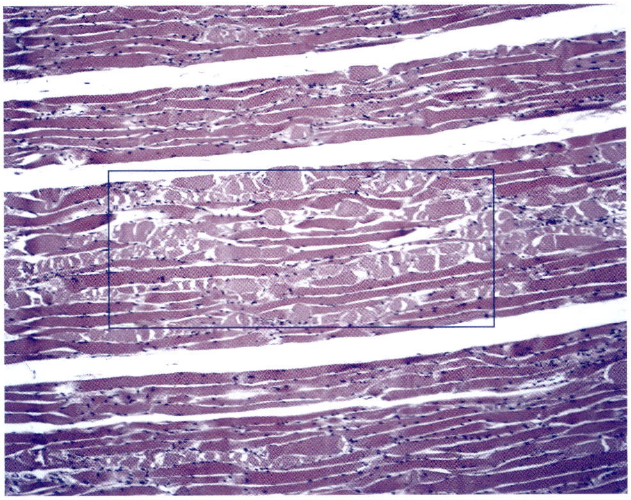

Figure 8.5: Pectoral muscle. Massive acute myodegeneration in a Gyr x Peregrine hybrid. Myodegeneration may occur after extensive exercise (hunting). HE stain.

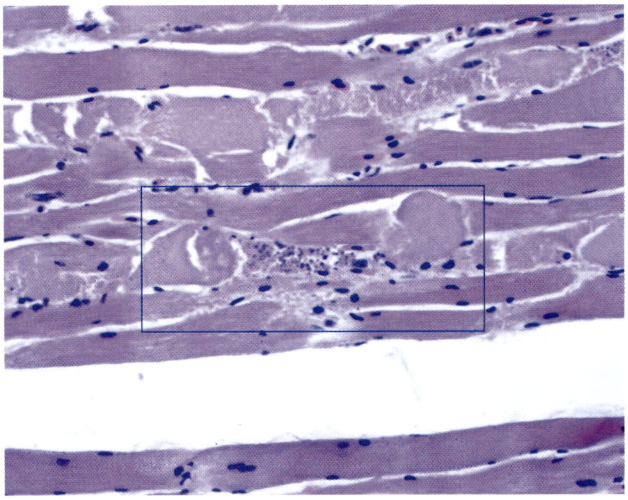

Figure 8.6: Higher magnification of Figure 8.5. Numerous swollen, pale fibres showing hyper contracted hyaline segments and floccular-degeneration. In such acute cases no inflammation is seen. HE stain.

Liver

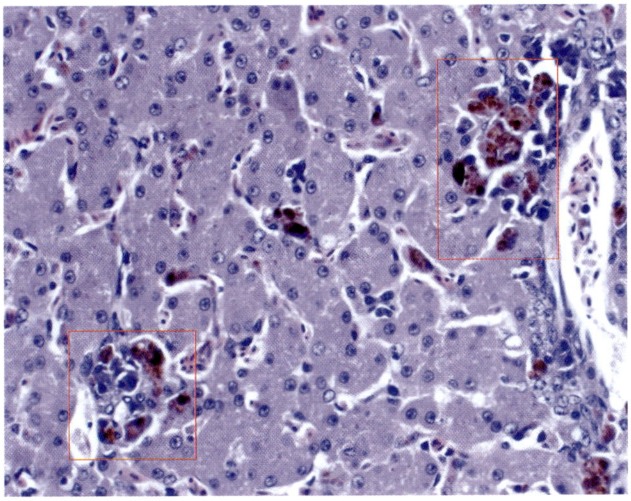

Figure 8.7. Hepatic haemochromatosis in a Gyr falcon. Marked accumulation of haemosiderin in Kupffer cells forming small granulomas. To a certain extent this is a normal finding. Severe haemosiderosis in falcon may be linked with concurrent infectious diseases.

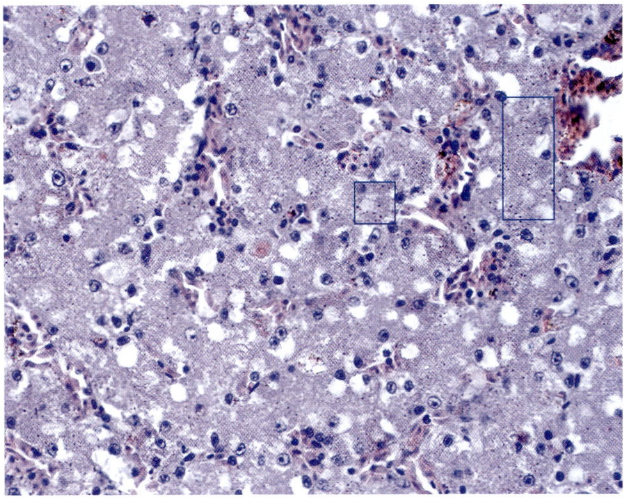

Figure 8.8: Hepatic haemochromatosis in a Gyr x Peregrine hybrid. Numerous hepatocytes containing small golden brown granulas of heamosiderin-pigment. In contrast to iron storage disease of some avian species, haemosiderin accumulation in hepatocytes is rare and always linked with accumulation in Kupffer cells.

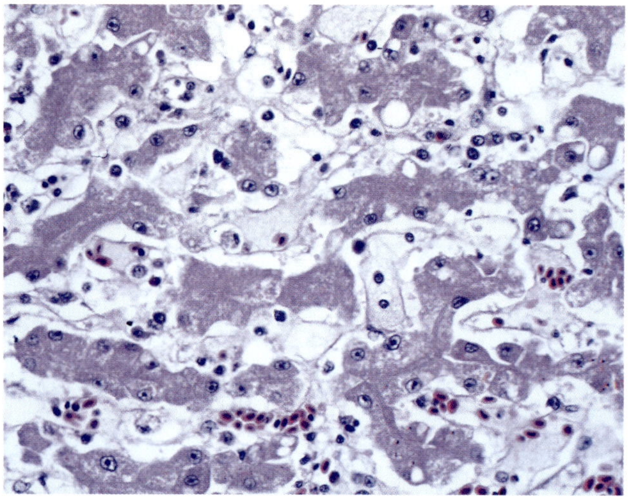

Figure 8.9: Liver. Massive oedema of the Disse's space in a Gyr falcon causing atrophy of the hepatocytic sheets. This lesions is usually linked with cardiovascular problems. HE stain.

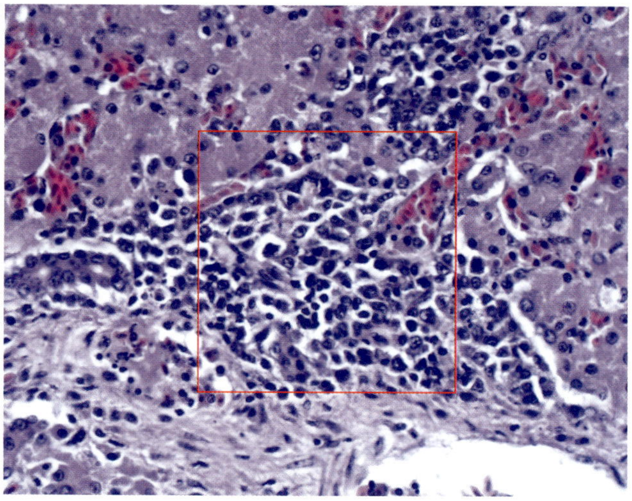

Figure 8.10: Interstitial hepatitis. Accumulation of mononuclear cells next to a Glisson's triangle. This lesion is very often found to a low extent, and most probably results from a previous acute inflammatory response. HE stain.

Chapter 9

Vaccination Regime

Very little is known about the efficacy of vaccines in *Falconidae*. So far no vaccines have been officially approved for use in falcons. However, we recommend the following vaccination programme for viral, bacterial and fungal diseases.

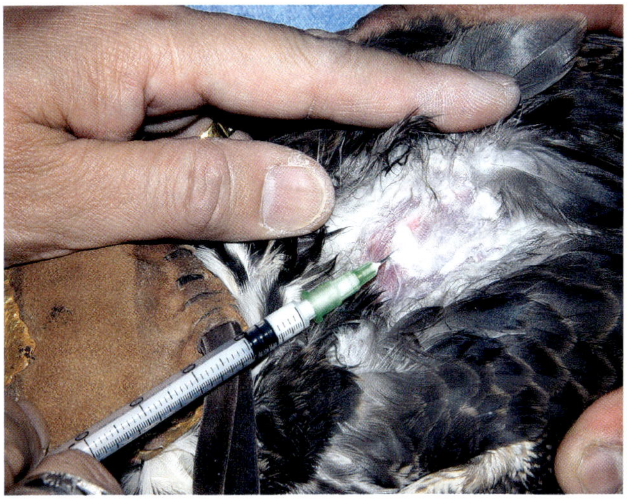

Figure 9.1: A Saker falcon is subcutaneously vaccinated into the neck with a PMV-1 vaccine.

Table 9.1: Vaccination programme for falcons

Disease	Vaccine	1st vaccination	Booster	Repeated Vaccination	Particularities
Pox	Live attenuated	6–9 weeks	After 4 weeks	Annually?	ADFA Abu Dhabi Falconpox Vaccine
Paramyxo	Inactivated oil adjuvant	6–9 weeks	After 4 weeks	Annually?	DuFaPA, 4 strains Dubai Falcon Paramyxovirus Vaccine
Herpes	Live attenuated	6–9 weeks	After 4 weeks	Annually?	DuFaHe Dubai Herpesvirus Vaccine
Clostridiosis	Inactivated $Al(OH)_3$ toxoid	6–9 weeks	After 4 weeks	Annually?	Enterovac 4 *C. perfringens* A strains
Clostridiosis	Hyperimmune serum, 1–2 ml i.v	Acute disease	–	–	Produced in eggs against 4 strains
Salmonella	Live 4 x 10^6 cfu	4–6 weeks	After 3 weeks	Annually?	SalmovacF *S. typhimurium*
Chlamydophilosis	Inactivated *C. psittaci*	4–6 weeks	After 3 weeks	Annually?	In preparation
Aspergillosis	Inactivated toxoid plus spores	4–6 weeks	After 3 weeks	Annually?	In experimental phase

9

Literature

ALTMAN, R.B., S.L. CLUBB, G.M. DORRESTEIN and K. QUESENBERRY. 1997. Avian Medicine and Surgery. WB Saunders Co., Philadelphia

CAMBPELL, T.W. 1988. Avian hematology and cytology. Iowa State University Press, Ames

FELDMAN, B.F., J.G. ZINKL and NEMI C. JAIN. 2000. Schalm's veterinary hematology. Lippincott Williams and Wilkens

FUDGE, A.M. 2000. Laboratory Medicine. Avian and Exotic Pets. W. B. Saunders Company

HARVEY, J.W. 2001. Atlas of veterinary hematology. W. B. Saunders Company

HAWKEY, C.M. and T.B. DENNET. 1989. A colour atlas of comparative Veterinary haematology. Wolfe Publishing Limited

KANEKO, J.J. 1989. Clinical biochemistry of domestic animals. Academic Press., Inc.

KINNE, J. and U. WERNERY. 2001. Pasteurellosis in falcons. Falco Newsletter **19**, 21–22

LIERZ, M., R. SCHMIDT and M. RUNGE. 2002. Mycoplasma species isolated from falcons in the Middle East. Vet. Rec. **151**, 92–93

LUMEIJ, J.T., J.D. REMPLE, P.T. REDIG, M. LIERZ and J.E. COOPER 2000. Raptor Biomedicine III. Zoological Education Network, Florida, U.S.A.

SAMOUR, J.H. and M.-A. D'ALOIA. 1996. Blood chemistry of the saker falcon *(Falco cherrug)*. Avian Pathology **25**, 175–178

SAMOUR, J. 2000. Avian Medicine. Mosby

SAMOUR, J. H. and J. NALDO. 2001. Serratospiculiasis in captive falcons in the Middle East: A review. J. Avian Med. and Surgery **15** (1), 2–9

SAMOUR, J.H. 2000. *Pseudomonas aeruginosa* stomatitis as a sequel to trichomoniasis in captive saker falcons (*Falco cherrug*). J. Avian Med. and Surgery **14** (2), 113–117

SAMOUR, J.H. 2000. Supraorbital trichomoniasis infection in two saker falcons (*Falco cherrug*). Vet. Rec. **146**, 139–140

SAMOUR, J.H. and M. A. PEIRCE. 1996. *Babesia shortti* infection in a saker falcon (*Falco cherrug*). Vet. Rec. **139**, 167–168

SAMOUR, J.H. and J. NALDO. 2002. Diagnosis and therapeutic management of lead toxicosis in falcons in Saudi Arabia. J. Avian Med. and Surgery **16** (1), 16–20

SAMOUR, J.H., T.A. BAILEY and I.F. KEYMER. 1995. Use of ammonium chloride in falconry in the Middle East. Vet. Rec. **137**, 269–270

THRALL, M.A. 2004. Veterinary hematology and clinical chemistry. Lippincott Williams and Wilkens, Wolters Kluwer Company

Subject index